Loretta J. Bradley • Elaine Jarchow
Beth Robinson

All About Sex

The School Counselor's Guide to Handling Tough Adolescent Problems

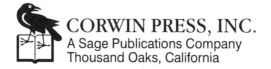
CORWIN PRESS, INC.
A Sage Publications Company
Thousand Oaks, California

For information:

Corwin Press, Inc.
A Sage Publications Company
2455 Teller Road
Thousand Oaks, California 91320
E-mail: order@corwinpress.com

SAGE Publications Ltd.
6 Bonhill Street
London EC2A 4PU
United Kingdom

SAGE Publications India Pvt, Ltd.
M-32 Market
Greater Kailash I
New Delhi 110 048 India

Printed in the United States of America

Library of Congress Cataloging-in-Publication Data

Bradley, Loretta J., 1941–
    All about sex: The school counselor's guide to handling tough adolescent problems / Loretta J. Bradley, Elaine Jarchow, Beth Robinson.
        p. cm. — (Practical skills for counselors)
    Includes bibliographical references and index.

    ISBN 0-8039-6692-X (cloth: acid-free paper)
    ISBN 0-8039-6693-8 (pbk.: acid-free paper)
    1. Teenagers—Sexual behavior. 2. High school students—Sexual behavior.
3. Junior high school students—Sexual behavior. 4. Educational counseling.
5. Counseling in secondary education. 6. Student counselors. 7. Sex instruction.
I. Jarchow, Elaine. II. Robinson, Beth. III. Title. IV. Series
    HQ27.B68 1999
    306.7'0835—dc21

                                                                98-040241

This book is printed on acid-free paper.

99 00 01 02 03 04 05 10 9 8 7 6 5 4 3 2 1

Production Editor: S. Marlene Head
Editorial Assistant: Kristen L. Gibson
Typesetter: Rebecca Evans
Cover Designer: Michelle Lee

Contents

Preface

All About Sex is designed to help school counselors respond to the challenging sexual issues of adolescence and understand the crucial role that sexual issues play in shaping teenagers' lives. Based on that understanding, it will help counselors translate knowledge into effective counseling interventions.

The three of us have raised teenagers and taught teenagers. Grappling with sexual issues is not a new task for us. We have each dealt with teen sexual issues in a variety of roles: parent, teacher, coach, counselor, and administrator. These roles have given us various perspectives on the issues that counselors face. Although we are considered competent professionals, we recognize that there are no easy answers to sexual issues or questions. We decided to explore these difficult issues with you because our experiences with teens have convinced us of the need to do so.

Unique Features

We selected topics we thought counselors would encounter frequently in a school setting. Knowing that we could not include all related topics, we focused on the most pertinent issues. We selected topics that met the following three criteria:

- The topic had to be related to sexual issues and popular enough to be of interest to junior and senior high school students.
- The topic had to be of interest to the counseling profession. Our guide for this area was presentations at recent counseling conferences and publications in counseling journals.
- The topic had to be one that would benefit students, enhance the school counselor's role in the school, and improve the school environment.

We have also approached problems honestly and have offered viable solutions. Case studies were used to augment our "solutions." We have even offered a menu of books and films for adolescents in the resource section.

Contents of the Book

In the first chapter, "Sexual Stuff: What's a School Counselor to Do?," we explain the purpose of the book. We introduce the topic of knowing the boundaries—school policies, parents, values and religion, and confidentiality. We present a series of case studies and answer common concerns counselors express in dealing with sexual issues.

In Chapter 2, "Coming of Age: Teenage Sexuality and Sexual Behavior," we look at such topics as adolescent insecurity, body image, sexuality, dating, identity exploration, sexual orientation, homophobia, and harassment. We suggest some helpful techniques for counselors to use to respond effectively to normal concerns teens have about sexuality.

In Chapter 3, "You Are Not Immune: Pregnancy and Sexually Transmitted Diseases," we consider teen pregnancy, contraceptives, HIV infection, and other diseases. Using a table on sexually transmitted diseases, we highlight symptoms, diagnosis, treatment, and prevention. We weigh the advantages and disadvantages of eight different birth control methods. Our case studies demonstrate a five-step assistance model. Several hands-on activities for students and parents are presented.

In Chapter 4, "This Isn't Supposed to Happen: Dealing With Sexual Violence," we suggest ways to help the counselor confidently respond to sexual abuse, incest, date rape, and stranger rape. We describe the symptoms alerting counselors of potential problems and present a disclosure dialogue. The differences in false and true allegations of sexual abuse are discussed. Real-world case studies demonstrate a six-step intervention model.

In Chapter 5, we provide a narrative account of how one counselor overcame her initial discomfort in responding to sexual issues of adolescents and developed effective prevention and intervention programs in her school. In addition, we explore the barriers and difficult situations counselors may encounter in addressing sexual issues with teens. We close the chapter by consolidating our conclusions and recommendations. We have also included suggested readings for counselors.

Acknowledgments

We appreciate the opportunity to contribute to Jeffrey Kottler's series, *Practical Skills for Counselors*. We want to thank Mrs. Kay Gleghorn for her assistance with preparing the manuscripts for Chapters 1, 3, 4, and 5; Dr. Holly Johnson for her suggestions regarding adolescent books and films; and Kitty Gage, Karla Hankins, Sally Larkins, Pat Leftwich, Keith Mask, Anita Reyna, Jerry Reyna, and John Sigle for their advice. We are grateful to the school counselors, teachers, parents, and teenagers who told us their stories, urged us to share those stories, and offered us advice. No doubt each older generation will continue to be amazed that the younger generation somehow thrives and survives.

Loretta J. Bradley
Elaine Jarchow
Beth Robinson
Lubbock, Texas

About the Authors

Loretta J. Bradley is Professor of Counselor Education and Chair of the Division of Educational Psychology and Leadership at Texas Tech University. She formerly was an Associate Professor of Human Development Counseling at Peabody College of Vanderbilt University and an Assistant Dean, College of Education at Temple University. Bradley earned her PhD at Purdue University. She is a licensed professional counselor (LPC), a licensed marriage and family therapist (LMFT), and an approved LPC supervisor and a LMFT supervisor.

Bradley is the President of the American Counseling Association (ACA) and a Past President of the Association for Counselor Education and Supervision (ACES). She has been the recipient of the following awards/honors: 1998 Fellow of the Salzburg Institute; 1996 President's Excellence in Teaching Award; 1995 COE Nominee for the Barney E. Rushing, Jr. Research Award; 1994 Texas Tech University nominee for Leadership Texas; 1993 COE Nominee for the President's Achievement Award; and 1992 and 1991 COE Nominee for the Barney E. Rushing, Jr. Research Award. In 1990, Dr. Bradley received the ACES Publication Award for her book, *Counselor Supervision: Principles, Process, and Practice,* and in 1987 she was the corecipient of the American Counseling Association's Research Award, an award representing an organization with more than 59,000 members.

Bradley has served as a member of the editorial boards of the *American Counselor* (Chair), *Counselor Education and Supervision Journal*, *Journal of Counseling and Development*, *Journal of Humanistic Education and Development*, and *Counseling and Human Development*. In addition to giving more than 100 presentations at professional meetings, she has authored or coauthored five books and more than 60 manuscripts and book chapters.

Elaine Jarchow is Dean of the College of Education at Texas Tech University. She holds degrees from Ohio University and Kent State University. Her major research area is international education, specifically curriculum decision making in emerging democracies and cultural awareness in international student teaching and faculty exchange settings. She is the author of more than fifty manuscripts, more than fifty conference presentations, and eighteen funded grants. She is coeditor of a 1996 book entitled, *Preparing Teachers to Teach Global Perspectives: A Handbook for Teacher Education* (Corwin Press). She chairs the American Association of Colleges for Teacher Education's Committee on International Education and is a member of the Association of Teacher Educators' International Affairs Committee, Global Education Task Force, and Publications Committee.

Beth Robinson is Assistant Professor in the Department of Behavioral Sciences at Lubbock Christian University and is an adjunct faculty member in the Division of Educational Leadership and Psychology at Texas Tech University. In addition to teaching, she counsels children and adolescents at the Children's Home of Lubbock. She is a Certified School Counselor and a Licensed Professional Counselor. Dr. Robinson completed her doctorate at Texas Tech University and her masters at West Texas A&M University. She is a frequent publisher and presenter at national and international conferences. Her research interests include multicultural issues in counseling and counseling with children and adolescents.

1

Sexual Stuff: What's a School Counselor to Do?

Lynn Adams couldn't wait to become a school counselor. After 4 years of teaching high school English, she was convinced that her students trusted her and sought her advice. She entered the school counseling program at a local university and completed the program in 2 years. Her first assignment was a metropolitan high school with 1,500 students. One of three counselors, she especially enjoyed helping college-bound students plan for their future. She also liked to solve a discipline problem or two. However, the "sex stuff" was especially troublesome. She looked back on the past 2 weeks and reviewed her notes. Six different teens described their problems as follows:

AUTHORS' NOTE: The authors have changed the names and identifying information in case studies in this book. Many of the case studies combine details from more than one client.

"My girlfriend wants to have sex but I think we should wait. She says I'm scared. She's right—I am!"

"I'm pregnant. I can't tell my parents. Where can I get an abortion?"

"I'm gay. Do you think anyone will accept me if they know?"

"I asked my boyfriend to stop, but he didn't. Is that rape?"

"I've got herpes. What do I do? My parents and friends will desert me."

"My stepfather visits my bedroom as soon as mom leaves for work. She loves him; he's our meal ticket. What should I do?"

Lynn tried a variety of strategies with students and used individual counseling, group counseling, family nights, and peer counseling. Sometimes she thought that she made a difference in helping students deal with sexual issues, but mostly she wondered what she could do to be more effective. When she was honest with herself, she admitted that she was uncomfortable discussing sexual issues with teens. The "sexual stuff" even triggered some feelings of anxiety for Lynn as she recalled her own sexual experiences during adolescence and how little help her well-meaning parents had provided her. Lynn recognized that she would have to explore her own values concerning sexuality.

Many of Lynn's students discussed experiences far different from her own. They lived lives she only read about. Sexual issues had received minimal coverage in her graduate training. She worried that she might have to discuss subjects deemed inappropriate by parents or administrators. In fact, she often avoided sexual issues in counseling sessions, urging students to consult their parents or clergy. Yet she knew that counseling adolescents positively about sexual issues was extremely important in the larger context of their lives.

A Reality Check

Today's sexually active teenagers may as easily invite a friend over for an after-school shower as they might once have invited that friend to a soda shop. Many young women share the details of their sex lives with friends in such intimate detail as that once found in the all-male locker room. Sex on the first or second date can easily become the norm for teens who do not wish to be labeled as prudes. Of course, there are still teenagers who are exploring their sexuality through dating, kissing, and petting "just enough," and looking forward to college, healthy sexual boundaries, and making responsible decisions about sexuality. They just may not visit the counselor's office very often, but they are out there.

Accepting kids today may not always be easy. After all, they challenge conventional norms, experiment with dangerous drugs, use bad language, join gangs, and show disrespect . . . in short, a number of them are just like we were. Of course, there are young people who are easy to like; they come from good homes, get good grades, respect us. The trick, of course, is to accept all these kids and to write prescriptions that we hope work for their particular maladies. How exciting it would be if the counselor could arrive on the secondary-school scene, analyze sexual adolescent concerns, and set young people on the path to satisfying relationships that last forever!

In the real world, many young people are searching for answers to questions about their sexual lives. Although adolescence is a natural time of sexual exploration and development, students are still confused by their changing bodies and unpredictable emotions. In addition to normal adolescent development, increasing numbers of students are dealing with sexual abuse, sexual harassment, pregnancy, sexually transmitted diseases, and other sexual issues. Effective counselors cannot avoid addressing sexual concerns. In fact, how you relate to these adolescents and their concerns will certainly determine your success as a counselor.

Knowing the Policies

Before addressing sexual issues with students, it is imperative that you learn the school policies and procedures regarding sexual issues and that you adhere to them. Failure to do so can result in your dismissal and the loss of all the help you were trained to give. Let's visit a typical high school.

Paulo Sanchez was new to the district, although he was not new to counseling. He regarded himself as an extremely successful school counselor, especially in the "sex stuff" arena. When Benito Adame, a popular junior football player, stopped in after school, Paulo was eager to help. Benito and his girlfriend had just begun having sex; Benito was worried about an unwanted pregnancy. Paulo had heard this concern a thousand times, and he did not think twice before launching into a discussion of teen pregnancy and sexually transmitted diseases. He always concluded the session by providing the student with a box of condoms and a promise of future counseling sessions, and today was no exception. He wished Benito well. The following morning, Paulo was surprised to find a "Please see me" notice from the principal.

The approaches you as a counselor take to tough adolescent problems of a sexual nature must be consistent with school policies and procedures. For example, in a case like Paulo's you must know the "rules" regarding the distribution of condoms. A number of other questions would be useful to consider:

1. What is the law regarding sexual abuse?
2. What is the law regarding confidentiality? When must you tell the parents?
3. What are your responsibilities toward the school? What policies and procedures will guide you? What must you report?
4. Must you notify school authorities about a student who threatens a homosexual teen?
5. Can you recommend birth control pills? Condoms?
6. How should you handle a student's plan to abort?
7. Is abstinence the only birth control policy your school advocates?
8. Can you recommend a doctor to give an HIV test to a student?
9. Can you suggest that a student consider adoption over abortion?
10. Can you organize a Gay Teens Support Group?

11. Must you report suspected "date rape"?
12. Can you counsel a teen to leave an abusive relationship?

School policy manuals are frequently very specific about the way sexuality will be addressed in the school district. Policies may dictate that course materials or class presentations about human sexuality be selected by the school board. Frequently, school policies insist that abstinence be presented as the preferred choice of behavior for students and that more attention be given to abstinence from sexual activity than to any other behavior. Most school districts have policies on how contraception is presented and whether condoms can be distributed.

As you can see, knowing your school's policies is essential. In fact, you might have to take the lead and either draft needed policies for consideration or suggest revisions of existing policies. Paulo Sanchez's principal praised him for relating well to students but pointed out that the distribution of condoms was not allowed. Together Paulo and his principal redrafted several policies and even organized a "safe sex" speaker for an optional after-school session.

Exploring Personal Values

We once knew a counselor who told his clients that he didn't counsel homosexuals or those who had sex before marriage. As a school counselor, you may well have a religious or value-oriented position with respect to abortion and homosexuality, but young people won't come to you if they think you've written them off. We believe that tolerance must underscore your approaches.

Remember what it was like to grow up? You knew it all, and the adults knew so little. The teens you counsel with respect to sexual issues may well have very different beliefs from yours. We think you must reexamine your own beliefs, values, and views about a variety of sexual issues. Let's visit one of Paulo's colleagues.

Dave Streetman liked counseling elementary school kids, and after 3 years of doing so was transferred to the senior high school. His last appointment of the day convinced him that he should seek a return to elementary school. Paul Arnold, a senior honor student, had just shared the fact that he was a homosexual. Paul's questions were many: Should he tell his parents? What would his classmates say? Would he be teased by his classmates? Were there some books he could read? Dave asked Paul to return the following day. "What can I say?" Dave thought. Dave's religious upbringing caused him to view homosexuality as a sin. Yet, Paul didn't seem like a sinner; he seemed like a bright young man who accepted himself and needed some advice. What should that advice be?

Global educators urge that we engage in perspective-taking exercises to recognize that there are those who have profoundly different worldviews from our own. School counselors, too, must recognize that the teens they counsel have worldviews that are quite different from their own.

Some religions do teach that homosexuality is a sin. How will you handle this belief (a) if you share it, or (b) if it's different from your own? We remember a young woman in our seminar who sat through a class where gay professors and students told their stories, urged tolerance, and gave suggestions for meeting their needs. In the next class, our student admitted that she had been deeply moved, but she still had to go with church teaching—homosexuality is a sin. What pleased us was her conflict resolution—she planned to listen to gay teens, to remain nonjudgmental, and to put them in touch with adults who could help them more than she could. What more could we have asked?

We don't recommend that you change your values or your religious orientation, but we do think that you should engage in perspective taking and that you should know when to refer teens to persons who can truly help them. Dave Streetman, by the way, convinced Paul to go with him to a local gay rights counseling agency. Paul was able to find answers to many of his questions, and Dave became a much more knowledgeable counselor in terms of help and referrals.

Working With Parents

Nora Edwards, another colleague of Paulo Sanchez and a 10-year veteran of secondary school counseling, liked working with parents.

Her parent advisory committee was especially productive. Often parents met with teen groups to discuss teenage sexuality. She wasn't surprised when Mrs. Fox asked to chat after a meeting, but she was surprised by the tenor of the conversation. Mrs. Fox had spied on her teenage daughter, Rachel, by reading her journal. What concerned her was her daughter's notation that if she did become pregnant, she would seek an abortion without telling her parents. Mrs. Fox asked Nora Edwards to promise to call her immediately if such a scenario were to ever reach Nora's office. "Wow!" thought Nora. "What do I say now?"

Parents' rights have become a confusing issue for the courts. For example, Montana requires parental permission to tattoo minors. In Florida, parents believe that teachers should reveal confidences such as journal writings about use of illegal drugs and the practice of unsafe sex. California permits females under age 18 to get an abortion without parental approval. Counselors must have a clear understanding of parents' rights in their school setting.

School counselors will enhance their effectiveness and credibility when they develop collaborative partnerships with parents. Parents must certainly play a role in your approaches. What is your responsibility toward them? Will you form a parent advisory committee? Will the committee represent different points of view? How will you handle these different points of view?

We suggest that you do what Nora Edwards did. Start with a group of about 10 parents, being sure to include both moms and dads. An SES cross section would be helpful. Having a conservative-to-liberal continuum will make for lively discussions. As a first step, you should involve them in some contemporary book and film chats. These vicarious experiences free parents from discussing their own children and from setting policies prematurely.

As you and the parent advisory committee gain a comfort level, you can move into more sensitive issues. How do they want you to advise the sexually active teen? Do they know the school and legal policies which guide you? Are there different strokes for different folks? Of course, you won't always agree, but these parents will appreciate your attempts to help both them and their children.

Summary

Perhaps one of the most difficult issues in counseling teens is addressing sexual issues. Being competent in assisting adolescents with sexual issues requires that you understand school policies, examine personal values, and learn to work with parents. Although we don't have a "formula" for counselors (like Lynn Adams, who is struggling to find effective ways to assist adolescents with sexual concerns), we do believe counselors can develop effective strategies for assisting teens.

Counselors may have to live with the notion that their short-term suggestions may never result in long-term gains. Teens are focused on the present and often have difficulty considering the long-term consequences of their actions. Part of working with adolescents is understanding that the results of interventions today may not be seen for several years in the future. In many cases, because the results of interventions cannot be determined until teens reach adulthood, counselors have to live with uncertainty concerning their effectiveness. How wonderful, though, it would be to know that we made a difference—that we significantly reduced the number of teen pregnancies and cases of incest. We must learn to measure our successes realistically and to follow some clients into the future to see if short-term solutions really result in long-term successes.

2

Coming of Age: Teenage Sexuality and Sexual Behavior

As counselors, we cannot deal with students without dealing with their sexuality. It does not take more than 15 minutes of conversation with teenagers to recognize that sexuality is an integral part of a teen's self-concept and identity. If we ignore or discount sexual issues in teens' lives, we have lost an opportunity to make a significant impact.

We cannot begin to talk with students about sexual issues until we have some understanding of how new and exciting sexuality is for a teen. Take a moment to think back to when you were a teen. Imagine you can hear the music you listened to and can see the friends you hung out with when you were an adolescent. Remember those feelings of awkwardness about your body and your uncertainty about any-thing sexual. Recall how you untucked your shirt to hide an erection or how you worried that everyone would know that you were having your period. Wow! Brings up some pretty strong memories and emotions, doesn't it? Few of us would subject ourselves to those insecurities again.

Teenagers still experience those feelings of uncertainty and awk-wardness, but they face decisions about sexuality at a younger age. Today's youth mature earlier and move through adolescence more quickly than youth in previous generations. Teens are making deci-sions about engaging in sexual activity at younger ages and fre-quently have only limited knowledge about sexual activities with which to make those decisions.

On Being an Adolescent

If counselors are going to be effective in helping adolescents deal with their developing sexuality, they must understand the develop-mental issues of adolescence. Adolescence is an intense time of change. Teens experience changes in their bodies, in their way of thinking, and in their relationships with peers and parents. As a result of these changes, teens are self-absorbed and preoccupied with fig-uring out who they are becoming. One of the developmental tasks for teens is coming to terms with their own sexuality. Adolescents focus on these changes and cope with these developmental tasks in different ways, but all teens experience the developmental issues discussed in this chapter.

There's an Alien in My Body

Literally, teens feel at times as though there is an alien being in their bodies because of all the changes they experience. They are developing breasts, growing body hair, having wet dreams, experi-encing mood changes, and starting their menstrual cycle. Their bod-ies are changing so quickly and unpredictably that teens are astounded. The following quotes illustrate some common teen per-ceptions about changes in their bodies.

"There's this great-looking girl in my English class. Just watching her in class, I feel like I could come in my jeans."

"I used to be a good student. I never got in trouble. Now my parents get notices from the school all the time that I'm not doing my work or I'm failing a class. I try. I really do, but all I think about is my boyfriend."

"I won't even get up and walk to the teacher's desk if I need help with my homework because I'm afraid I'll get a hard-on."

"I hate my period. I feel awful all the time, and I start crying for no reason. Why did this happen to me?"

"It's like, all I think about is sex. I'll see a girl's bra strap and I won't be able to quit thinking about what it would be like to have sex with her."

As teens develop an interest in sexuality, they feel overwhelmed and a bit frightened by how their bodies respond when they are attracted to someone. Their bodies feel alien to them and they experience awkwardness when they don't understand how their bodies are changing.

Although all teens experience changes in their bodies, some teens experience changes earlier or later than their friends. Whether teens develop sexually earlier or later than their friends, it causes them stress and distress. If a girl has smaller breasts than her friends, she wonders if anyone will ever ask her out on a date. If a teen gets an erection 15 times a day, and his friend gets an erection 6 times a day, he wonders if he is a "pervert." Being different from everyone else can be interpreted by teens as being weird or disgusting.

I'm on Center Stage

All teens experience the developmental challenge of believing that they are being watched by everyone else. Teens feel as though they are on center stage in Carnegie Hall with a spotlight focused on them every minute of the day. Because teens believe everyone is watching them and critiquing how they dress and what they do, they feel pressure to look perfect and to conform to their peers' expectations.

Imagine how the concern of being on center stage affects a teenager when her breasts begin to develop. She believes everyone in the room will turn and look at her as though she is the center of attention. Guess what she thinks they are looking at? Her breasts, of course. She worries that her breasts are too small or too large. She wonders if her nipples show through her shirt or if her breasts shake when she runs.

Similarly, consider how a teenager feels when he is required to shower in a locker room. He feels self-conscious about being naked in a locker room with his peers because he thinks everyone will be looking at his penis. He worries that his penis is smaller than his peers' and that he won't be satisfactory as a sexual partner. When he experiences an erection in the locker room, he is concerned that his peers will assume that he is gay.

Because teens feel that everyone is watching them, they experience tremendous anxiety about normal development and social situations. They perceive that other people will be scrutinizing their interactions with peers and their sexual development.

Picture Perfect

Because of changes in the way teenagers think, they are able for the first time to conceptualize what is ideal. Suddenly, teens are comparing themselves and everyone else with an "ideal" or perfect standard. Frequently, teens look for boyfriends or girlfriends that have "ideal" bodies or personalities; they believe they, too, should have perfect bodies.

If you've ever tried to share a bathroom with a teenager in the morning, you understand how important the "perfect" look can be. Access to the bathroom may be blocked for hours as teens scrutinize their faces, hair, and bodies for extended periods of time before appearing in public. They struggle to camouflage pimples, get their teeth pearly white, and to find a scent that pleasantly distinguishes them. Ironically, teens seem to want the physical attributes they do not possess. For example, some teens labor to straighten their curly hair, while other teens work to curl their straight hair. All of these morning rituals occur in the pursuit of perfection.

A glimpse into a high school weight room will only convince you that this quest for perfection extends beyond facial and follicle transformations. Teens sweat to create a more perfect body by lifting, curling, and pressing different types of weights. They expend energy running, biking, and doing sit-ups in hopes they will lose or gain inches in different parts of their bodies. Frequently, they augment these fitness pursuits with dieting to help them reach an "ideal" body image.

Who Am I Today?

Although teens don't consciously decide who they want to be every day, identity exploration and formation is one of the most important developmental tasks of adolescence. Teenagers search for ways to fit in with their peers and become more independent from their parents. They frequently change clothing, hairstyles, and even types of friends as they try to decide who they want to be. In addition, they may want to announce who they are by wearing strikingly different clothing or by having a tattoo displayed that represents part of their identity.

Part of teen's identity exploration and formation involves integrating their sexuality into their self-concept. An initial step in integrating sexuality into self-concept is exploring cultural beliefs about sexuality. Counselors recognize that sexuality issues are not viewed the same way in all cultures. Specific issues to explore with teens that affect identity formation include the following:

■ How do family members view dating?

■ How does being male or female influence the rules that your family places on dating, curfew, drinking, and socializing?

■ How do members of your racial/ethnic group view sexuality among adolescents?

■ Are the rules the same for young men and women?

■ What do the members of your racial/ethnic group say about sexual intimacy before marriage?

■ Does your spirituality influence your views of sexuality?

Once teens have explored their culture's beliefs and values about sexuality, they can integrate sexuality into their self-concept by clarifying their own beliefs and values about sexuality. In clarifying what they believe, teens set a foundation for making healthy and responsible decisions about their own sexuality.

After exploring cultural values about sexuality, teens may intentionally make choices that clash with their family's cultural values as a way of distinguishing their own personal identity. A teenager raised in a conservative religious home with parents who oppose abortion may participate in a pro-choice organization, or a teenager whose parents have actively supported condom distribution in schools may voice the belief that abstinence should be advocated rather than birth control. These "rebellions" are part of the developmental process of establishing a clear personal identity and are generally transient.

Where's the Instruction Manual?

Because teens don't have previous experiences to guide them in making decisions about dating and sex, they certainly might benefit from an instruction manual to guide them through decisions about these issues. As teens develop sexually, everything is a new experience: first wet dream, first kiss, first party, first love. The novelty of all these experiences contributes to the intensity of teen responses because they can't compare their current feelings and experiences with any other experiences. Teens anticipate dating, but often experience anxiety when they are asked out on a date because they don't know what is expected in dating situations.

Imagine that an attractive teen walks into your office. She sits and fidgets in her chair as she twirls her hair in her hand. Finally she glances up at you and says, "I think there is something wrong with me."

You are puzzled because this student doesn't have problems in school and seems to interact well with her classmates.

"Tell me what you mean."

"Something's wrong with me. I've been dating Abdul for a couple of weeks and I'm getting sick all the time."

As a counselor, the first option you consider is that the client is pregnant and is experiencing morning sickness.

"When are you getting sick?"

"Just when we go out."

Mentally, you cross pregnancy off the list of possibilities and consider anxiety as an option.

"Are you nervous about dating Abdul?"

"I was the first time we went out, but I like him a lot and we have a lot of fun."

"Tell me a little more about what happens when you get sick."

"Well, I don't actually throw up, but I feel like I'm going to be sick. I know something awful is wrong with me." The student hesitates for a minute. She looks down at the floor and lets her hair fall to cover her face, "It's just that . . . hmm . . . every time Abdul kisses me, my stomach feels sick. I know it's weird. Nobody else gets sick when they kiss guys. What's wrong with me?"

There was nothing "wrong" with this teen. She was experiencing a normal response to being kissed by her boyfriend. When she became sexually aroused while kissing her boyfriend, the only prior experience she had that was similar to the physical response was when she would get anxious and become nauseous. She connected her physical response with nausea because she had no prior experience with being sexually aroused. She was quite relieved when her counselor explained that she was experiencing a normal sexual response and there wasn't anything "wrong" with her.

The World of Adolescents

In addition to understanding the developmental tasks of adolescents, counselors also need to understand the world adolescents live in today. Through music, television, movies, and pornography, teens are exposed to models of sexuality that can be aggressive, degrading, and removed from the context of a relationship. They get mixed messages about sexuality. For example, they may be told that sex is a special union between two people who are married. At the same time, they see sex used to sell everything from coffee to clothes in the media. It should not be surprising that teens seem to be confused about love, sex, and popularity. Because students have little sense of sexuality in the context of relationships, decisions about sex don't consider personal values or long-term goals.

Similarly, students experience a curriculum at school that sends mixed messages because sex is taught in both the classroom and in the halls of schools. In the classrooms, students learn about anatomy, sexually transmitted diseases, and pregnancy. What students don't learn in the classroom is how sex is part of a relationship with another person and how sexual activities may have emotional as well as physical consequences. Classrooms don't teach students how to interact with their peers or how to set healthy sexual boundaries. As a result, students have difficulty translating what they learn in the classroom to what they do on a date. Felicia, an eighth grader, went to see her school counselor because she was afraid that she might be pregnant because she had oral sex. She believed the only way she could get pregnant was by swallowing sperm so it would go into her stomach. Felicia was unable to connect what she had learned in the classroom with the sexual experiences of her own life.

In the hallways of the school, being sexually active is viewed as a rite of passage to adulthood. As a result, students feel pressured to be sexually active without concern for the context of a meaningful relationship. Teens may have sex with peers they hardly know and may not recognize the dangers of engaging in sexual activities with strangers. For example, Amanda, a 14-year-old, attended a church youth group activity. At that youth activity, she met Randy for the first time. Randy asked her to go out to his car and have sex with him. She agreed. They had sex and then returned to the youth group meeting a little later. Several weeks later, Amanda told her youth minister about having sex with Randy. Amanda was stunned at the youth minister's reaction. She had expected a lecture on waiting until she was married to have sex. Instead, the youth minister focused on how dangerous it was for her to get in a car with someone she didn't know. Amanda had never considered the danger of the situation. All she had been concerned about was whether Randy would like her. Amanda is representative of teens who find it difficult to resist engaging in sexual activities because they are seeking peer approval and who have little understanding of sex as part of a relationship.

Sexual Orientation

In the midst of the turmoil of adolescent development, it is not surprising that students struggle with issues of sexual orientation. John Forbes knew he was gay by the time he was 14 years old. He hid this fact from his family and friends until he was a high school senior. At the beginning of his senior year, John's school hired a new counselor, Mr. Dexter. Because Mr. Dexter appeared to be both understanding and caring, John decided to divulge his secret and to ask for help.

Alex Dexter brought a wealth of experience to his new assignment. He knew that adolescence was frequently a time when individuals were coming to terms with sexual orientation. Mr. Dexter had counseled a number of lonely, isolated male and female teens who were either confused by issues of sexual orientation or who identified themselves as gay or lesbian. He even remembered working with homophobic counselors and teachers. Sadly, he also attended the funerals of two gay teens who committed suicide. When John Forbes unburdened himself, Alex Dexter was ready to help.

John began their first counseling session with a rambling narrative about himself. Before he acknowledged his homosexuality, he recognized that he was different from his peers. While other elementary school students struggled with mathematics and reading, John also wrestled with determining who he was. During his middle school years, he recalled students using words such as "fruitcake," "faggot," and "queer," and he not only worried that coming out would result in a loss of friends, but in addition he feared further ridicule and physical assault. He found it easier to laugh than object when his friends stereotyped homosexuals.

During the early years of senior high school, John knew that he wanted to experiment with a gay relationship. He worried, however, about AIDS and the guilt he might feel. During a family vacation, John entered into a sexual relationship with a young man he knew he would never see again. Lately, he wondered if the future would hold positive, fulfilling relationships that he could share with family and friends.

Alex Dexter assisted John as he confronted his many questions and concerns. Initially, Alex recommended that John read personal narratives by other teens and discuss them with him. At other times, they worked on defining healthy sexual and relationship boundaries for John. Alex also helped John open up to his parents and friends and deal with their reactions toward him. At the end of John's senior year, Alex helped him develop a support network in community agencies and discussed John's plans for the future.

Alex Dexter was prepared to deal with the issues and unique challenges counselors face when counseling gay and lesbian youth. In order to be effective in counseling gay or lesbian adolescents or adolescents who are confused about their sexual orientation, counselors must first be willing to examine and confront their own issues and concerns about sexual orientation and homosexuality.

Very few counselors come to sessions about gay and lesbian youth without a certain level of discomfort. At a recent national convention for teacher educators, the sessions on gay and lesbian youth were well attended, but some conference attendees admitted that they felt uncomfortable among the gay and lesbian presenters, that they worried about being labeled as too liberal, and that they couldn't in any way accept alternative lifestyles.

Each counselor should embark on a voyage of discovery—attending conference sessions that deal with gay and lesbian issues, reading about homosexuality, visiting with gays and lesbians and homosexual advocacy groups, seeking out community resources, and talking with successful counselors of gay and lesbian youth. A voyage of self-discovery can often be painful. Sometimes we still feel inadequate to face difficult challenges. One of our students sat through a class on counseling gay and lesbian youth. She visited with gay students and faculty and read numerous personal narratives. At the end of the course, she still held fast to her religious belief that homosexuality is a sin, but she recognized that her understanding had grown and that she could help gay and lesbian youth find professional counselors to assist them.

Confusion About Sexual Orientation

Although sexual orientation is frequently conceptualized in the discrete categories of homosexual or heterosexual, counseling issues highlight the need for a broad conceptualization of sexual orientation. Walter, a junior in high school, began to stop by Clarissa Washington's counseling office 2 or 3 times a week. He would visit with Clarissa for a few minutes and then leave. Every time Walter stopped by Clarissa's office, he was trying to work up the courage to ask a question.

One afternoon, Walter finally blurted out, "How would a guy know if he's gay?"

Clarissa wants to know what Walter's concerns are, so she responds, "Walter, tell me how you think a guy would know if he is homosexual?"

"Uh, I guess if he had sex with another guy."

"Would a guy be homosexual if he had sex with girls a lot of times and only had sex with a guy one time?"

"I don't know. Maybe not. Maybe he did it with a guy, but liked doing it with girls better. I guess he wouldn't be gay if he liked doing it with girls better, would he?"

Clarissa words her responses carefully in interacting with Walter because she knows that during sexual exploration, children and teens can engage in sexual activities with someone of the same gender, yet still be attracted to individuals of the opposite gender. Clarissa continues her conversation with Walter and explains that sexual behavior generally occurs across a continuum (see Figure 2.1). She goes on to explain that people can have sexual experiences with individuals of the same gender or be sexually abused by individuals of the same gender, but be heterosexual. She also explains that bisexual individuals engage in both heterosexual and homosexual behavior.

Walter is representative of adolescents who are confused about sexual orientation. Teens who have experienced sexual abuse, particularly by individuals of the same gender, may believe that the abuse defines their sexual orientation. Similarly, adolescents who have engaged in exploration or experimentation may mistakenly believe that the experience defines their sexual orientation. Counselors can assist students by helping them recognize that sexual orientation involves attraction and affection as well as sexual activity. In exploring sexual orientation issues, it is important that counselors remain supportive and accepting of students. If counselors directly

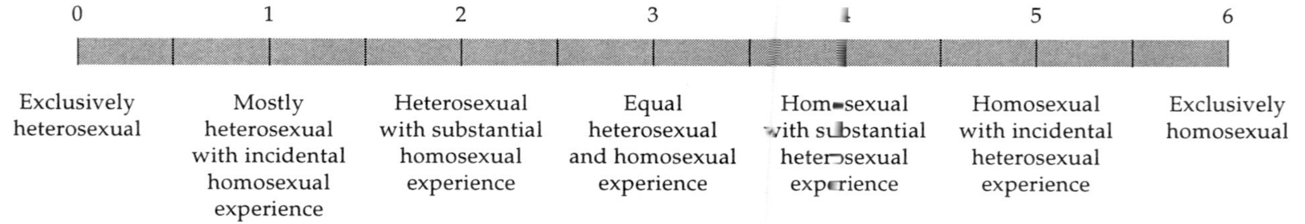

Figure 2.1. Continuum of Sexual Behavior

0	1	2	3	4	5	6
Exclusively heterosexual	Mostly heterosexual with incidental homosexual experience	Heterosexual with substantial homosexual experience	Equal heterosexual and homosexual experience	Homosexual with substantial heterosexual experience	Homosexual with incidental heterosexual experience	Exclusively homosexual

or indirectly communicate that only being heterosexual is acceptable, students will seek information from someone else.

Homophobia

In many schools, students who are gay or lesbian face harassment and, in some cases, physical assault. Homophobia contributes to hostility toward gays and lesbians. Homophobia is an unrealistic fear of, or a negative attitude toward, gays and lesbians. Gays and lesbians are often targets of homophobia. In a homophobic society, males are punished for "feminine behaviors," and females are punished for "masculine" behaviors. Homophobia contributes to stigmatization of gay and lesbian students and a restriction of opportunities for these students. Homophobia may result in inadequate and harmful counseling interventions for gay and lesbian adolescents. Ethics require that counselors be aware of their own attitudes about homosexuality and make referrals to another counselor when necessary.

Specific Interventions

In addition to the general approaches discussed in this book, counselors can assist gay and lesbian teens by using the following strategies:

1. Student and Staff Development

A crucial task for counselors is providing professional development for both students and staff to address homophobia. Staff and student development must emphasize that gay and lesbian youth have the right to receive their education in a safe and secure environment. Ideally, effective staff and student development will assist gay and lesbian youth in forming relationships with some nonjudgmental and caring peers, staff, and teachers.

The counselor must be prepared to provide training for all staff members—administrators, teachers, secretaries, cafeteria workers, custodians, bus drivers. Eliminating homophobia is a difficult task, and involving everyone in the workplace is important. Gay and lesbian staff, students, and parents can serve as consultants and role models. Providing opportunities to visit community agencies that serve gay and lesbian youth will add to the staff's understanding.

During staff development, counselors can emphasize the importance of having curriculum materials that avoid stereotypes and provide accurate portrayals of gays and lesbians. Certainly, the curriculum should reinforce the idea that families in which a parent is gay or lesbian are okay families. The curriculum need not glorify these individuals but should make note of their positive contributions to our society.

Student development activities are more difficult to plan. Adults usually receive staff development with a degree of respect; students may resent the approaches, laugh and ridicule the presenters, and remain largely unchanged in their behavior. The counselor and administrators must first work on cultivating an atmosphere of respect, acceptance, and caring—the very heart of multiculturalism. A program that infuses tolerance throughout the curriculum is essential. Many activities in our resource section can be explored to plan a series of meaningful student development activities.

2. Parent Outreach

Ann Todd's parents gave her everything within their means—love, understanding, and support. Mrs. Todd was a nurse at the local hospital, and Mr. Todd was an accountant for a large firm. Summer vacations were spent at a nearby lake cabin. Ann received a late-model used car for her 16th birthday. A year later, on her 17th birthday, Ann gave her parents a very unexpected announcement—she told them she was a lesbian. The Todds reacted with shock and dismay. Surely, Ann was mistaken, they thought. After several months of intense family counseling, the Todds not only accepted their daughter but also offered to assist other gay and lesbian teens and their families. The Todds are not unique in their initial reactions to their daughter's announcement, but they are unique in their early acceptance and decision to help others. Although school counselors cannot hope for too many parents like the Todds, they can cultivate and learn from such parents.

In contrast to the Todds, some parents may be angry with their children and refuse to acknowledge their homosexuality or, worse yet, reject their child because of his or her homosexuality. Parents need support and assistance when learning of their child's homosexuality. The school counselor should consider recommending family therapy and referrals to organizations such as Parents and Friends of Lesbians and Gays (P-FLAG). Some parents will move along the continuum of acceptance to advocacy while others will do well to accept their teens. As counselors, we must recognize that these parents need time to work through feelings that are new and frightening to them.

3. Support Services

Gay and lesbian teens are often lonely and frightened and benefit greatly from establishing connections with individuals of the same sexual orientation. Counselors need to be aware of available support groups and local agencies that offer assistance for gay and lesbian teens. In addition, counselors can provide access to gay- and lesbian-sensitive literature and involve community agencies in their staff development programs.

4. Advocacy

Becoming an advocate for gay and lesbian youth may involve more risk taking than some counselors wish to undertake. At one end of the advocacy continuum are such activities as providing gay and lesbian youth with adequate reading materials or planning school assemblies with gay and lesbian speakers. At the other end of the continuum, however, are such activities as ensuring that school policies and procedures protect the rights of gay and lesbian youth and punish those students who persecute them. In addition, counselors can consult with the school board and area legislators to develop policies that eliminate unfair hiring practices.

Help Is on the Way

Counselors can use an understanding of adolescent developmental issues and the following general guidelines to respond effectively to teens who are experiencing normal developmental concerns.

1. *Normalize experiences.* Teens do not have previous experience with how their bodies are developing and responding; therefore, they do not have any standard of comparison. One of the most beneficial interventions a counselor can provide is to normalize the experience for teens. The counselor can ease teens' concerns about their developing bodies by explaining to them that all teens experience the same thing and that adults have gone through adolescence and experienced the same concerns. Teens may not know that most males experience wet dreams and get hard-ons when they are attracted to someone during adolescence. Similarly, females may not know that many women have concerns about pelvic exams and have to learn how to use tampons. Generally, information about how our bodies respond when we are sexually aroused and how our bodies change during adolescence will help normalize the experience for teens.

2. *Use natural opportunities for interaction.* Although classroom guidance activities and structured support groups may be effective for presenting general information about sexuality to teens, it is the daily opportunities for interaction that will allow a counselor to establish a relationship with students. Counselors need to use casual interactions in the hallways, at extracurricular activities, or during lunch breaks to build relationships with teens. Teens are not going to talk with a stranger in an office if they have concerns about their developing sexuality. They need to feel comfortable with the counselor and they need to believe that the counselor is approachable. The only way to help teens feel comfortable is by interacting with them in nonthreatening situations. Effective counselors understand this and capitalize on opportunities to interact with students on their turf.

3. *Recognize "fishing" expeditions.* During casual interactions, teens will often "fish" for information from the counselor or other adults. They "fish" for information by indirectly verbalizing concerns they have about sexuality or other personal issues. They will not come out and directly approach the subject, but they will indirectly try to gain some information from the counselor. Students approach subjects indirectly because they are trying to decide whether to trust the school counselor. Teens may bring up a current news story or ask a counselor what he or she believes about an issue. For example, a counselor sees a student in the cafeteria at school.

Teen:	"Hey, Mr. Johnson! How's it goin'?"
Counselor:	"Things are goin' okay. How about with you?"
Teen:	"It's all right. You know something Mr. Johnson, I've got a question for you."
Counselor:	"What's your question?"
Teen:	"Well, my friends and I have been talking about movies and I just wondered if you would let your daughter watch an R-rated movie?"
Counselor:	"I don't know. I think it would depend on the movie. What do you think I should do?"

In this interaction, the counselor recognized that the student might be trying to "check out" the counselor's attitudes. One of the unstated concerns in the scenario about watching R-rated movies is that R-rated movies often depict sexually explicit situations. The teen asking the question may be indirectly asking if the counselor believes teens can handle sexual issues and experiences. If the counselor had given a firm negative answer, the teen might have assumed the counselor would not be willing to objectively explore the situation with her. The counselor in this scenario responded to the inquiry and opened the conversation up for the teen to express her views or concerns. If counselors recognize "fishing" expeditions like the one in this scenario and respond appropriately, they can communicate more effectively with teens.

4. *Encourage conversation.* Counselors can encourage teenagers to discuss sexual issues by listening attentively and being cautious about giving advice. Generally, teens will respond better to counselors who are providing information and who refrain from making critical or judgmental remarks concerning sexual issues. Without realizing it, counselors convey a negative attitude through a harsh or disapproving tone of voice or communicate indirectly that sex is "bad" or "dirty." Counselors should be aware of their own feelings and values about sexuality. Adolescents are sexual beings, and effective counselors accept teens' struggles with sexual concerns. With this awareness, counselors can more effectively monitor their own responses to teen concerns about sexuality. Counselors must diligently strive not to impose their values on clients. Rather, they should

encourage teen clients to explore and establish their own values concerning sexuality. Counselors who try to impose their values on their clients will often find teens are unwilling to discuss sexual issues with them because teens perceive that the counselor is lecturing rather than listening.

5. *Don't minimize teen experiences.* Counselors have the advantage of life experiences to help them place teen concerns in context. Counselors recognize that losing a boyfriend or feeling self-conscious about a changing body are part of adolescent development. Although this allows counselors to recognize that the intensity of feelings and the crisis created by developing sexuality will be resolved in time, teens do not have the luxury of this perspective. Teens won't be comforted by statements like "One day you'll laugh about this," or "You'll fall in love again and forget all about this girlfriend." Statements like this minimize the emotional intensity of adolescents. Effective interventions demand that counselors acknowledge and accept the intensity of teen emotions about sexuality.

Effective Techniques

In addition to the general guidelines counselors can use in discussing sexual development, there are several techniques counselors can use to help students make responsible decisions about their own sexuality. These techniques are proactive rather than reactive and can be used to help teens clarify their own values and find ways to respond to peer pressure.

Exploring Personal Concerns About Sexuality

Teens frequently have concerns about their own sexuality that they are unable to identify or unable to verbalize. Developing an effective strategy for assisting adolescents with sexual issues requires counselors to be able to identify the personal concerns teens have about their own sexuality. Counselors can obtain this information through informal conversations, but in some situations, counselors may want to conduct a quick assessment of teens' personal concerns

A = Almost Always *B* = Frequently *C* = Occasionally *D* = Seldom E = Almost Never					
1. I am confused by my own feelings about sexuality.	A	B	C	D	E
2. I dream about sex.	A	B	C	D	E
3. I think about sex.	A	B	C	D	E
4. I like my own body.	A	B	C	D	E
5. I don't know what sexual behavior is okay for me.	A	B	C	D	E
6. I make bad decisions about my own sexual behavior.	A	B	C	D	E
7. I engage in sexual activities without thinking about the consequences.	A	B	C	D	E
8. Sexual relationships are a hassle.	A	B	C	D	E
9. I think about sexual activities more than my peers.	A	B	C	D	E
10. When I am engaging in sexual activities, I get confused about my feelings.	A	B	C	D	E
11. I have sexual urges and don't know what to do.	A	B	C	D	E
12. I engage in sexual activities without thinking about anyone except myself.	A	B	C	D	E
13. I get good feelings in my body when I think about sex.	A	B	C	D	E
14. Teenagers should be able to do anything they want sexually.	A	B	C	D	E
15. A woman has the right to say "no" to sex with a man.	A	B	C	D	E
16. It is okay for kids to touch themselves in their private parts.	A	B	C	D	E
17. A sexual relationship between two people of the same sex is okay.	A	B	C	D	E
18. Two people should care about each other before they engage in sexual activities.	A	B	C	D	E
19. If a woman doesn't want to have a baby, she should choose to have an abortion.	A	B	C	D	E

Exhibit 2.1. Questionnaire: Exploring Personal Concerns About Sexuality

about sexuality. Exhibit 2.1 is provided as a tool to help counselors identify these concerns about sexuality and begin to talk with teens about these issues.

Know How Far Is Far Enough

Deciding how far is far enough is a dilemma every teen faces. As teens decide if they are going to participate in different types of sexual activities, they may have a variety of questions.

Is it all right to kiss on my first date?

Is it wrong to get into petting or necking?

Am I weird if I masturbate?

Is oral sex wrong?

Is it okay to do everything except go "all the way?"

When am I old enough?

Counselors can help teens address their concerns about "how far is far enough" by assisting teens in clarifying why they would choose to engage in a sexual activity. For example, Mary has been dating Ben for 2 months. Ben has a driver's license and on several occasions has driven to an isolated place and parked the car. Mary initially enjoyed "making out" with Ben, but she reports to her counselor that she feels uncomfortable now when she and Ben go out on dates. Mary states, "We've been making out, kissing and stuff, but I know what comes next. I know I should want to have sex, but I don't know if I'm ready for sex."

A counselor could assist Mary by helping her clarify the reasons why she would or would not choose to engage in intercourse. As she considers why she wouldn't engage in intercourse, Mary might express concerns about pregnancy and sexually transmitted diseases or she might even state that she's not sure she loves Ben. On the other hand, she might verbalize the fact that sex could be fun and all her friends are having sex as reasons to engage in intercourse with Ben. Once Mary indicated why she would engage in intercourse, the counselor could help her consider whether she felt those reasons were sufficient for deciding to engage in intercourse, or if she had some other criteria she believed were necessary before making a decision to engage in intercourse.

Counselors can use group activities to help teens clarify their own sexual values and to decide what boundaries they want to set for themselves. For example, a counselor can write the following questions on note cards. The note cards can be shuffled and stacked or can be placed in a large container. The participants in the group take turns drawing a note card and answering the question on the note card. Once the participant who drew the question answers it, the other participants can discuss their responses to the question.

1. How old should a person be to start dating? Are there different rules for boys and girls?
2. How old should a person be when he or she has intercourse for the first time? Are there different rules for boys and girls?
3. What is a good age for a person to become a parent?
4. Is sex good, bad, or in between? Why?
5. How should two people decide if they are going to have a sexual relationship?
6. If a man doesn't want to use birth control, but the woman doesn't want to get pregnant, what should happen?
7. Is abortion okay? Who should decide if a woman gets an abortion?
8. When is sexual behavior abusive?
9. What is sexual harassment?
10. What does your religion teach about sex?
11. What are your parents' beliefs about sex?
12. What do you think about pornography?

Reverse the Pressure

Frequently, teens experience pressure to engage in sexual activities before they are ready to make these decisions. They have boyfriends or girlfriends who say things like the following:

"If you really loved me, you would have sex with me."

"If you really cared about me, you wouldn't tell me no."

"If you don't have sex with me, I'll find someone who will."

"Everyone else is doing it."

Counselors can help teens learn to reverse the pressure. Teens can turn around statements intended to pressure them into engaging in sexual activities. Examples of ways to reverse the pressure are the following:

"If you really loved me, you wouldn't pressure me to have sex with you."

"Show me you care about me by not pushing me into having sex with you."

"Go ahead and find someone else to have sex with you."

"If everybody else is doing it, you shouldn't have any trouble finding someone else."

Counselors can help teens develop their ability to reverse the pressure by using role-playing in group activities. The counselor can assume the role of the individual pressuring a teen to have sex. Group participants can be encouraged to "coach" the counselor by telling the counselor what to say and how to act. Teens in the group are then given the opportunity to respond to the pressure. Initially, students generally respond in a timid fashion, but the exercise can be repeated until group participants can assertively reverse the pressure.

Don't Pressure Others

In addition to recognizing that they can reverse the pressure to engage in sexual activities, teens need to recognize when they are pressuring someone else to participate in sexual activities. Pressuring others involves both directly pressuring a boyfriend or girlfriend to engage in sexual activities or indirectly pressuring peers by trying to embarrass or humiliate teens who aren't engaging in sexual activities. Counselors can help teens recognize that everyone develops and matures differently, and that this developmental process affects when someone is ready to participate in sexual activities. The following questions can be used in group activities to help students recognize when coercion occurs in making decisions about sexual activities.

1. Do both participants understand and agree to what they are going to do before they start?
2. Does one participant make all the decisions?
3. Does one partner have an idea and badger the other partner into doing it?
4. What happens if one partner decides to stop?
5. Are bribes or threats used?
6. Does one partner engage in a sexual behavior only because he or she is afraid?
7. Is engaging in sexual behavior used as an initiation into a group?

It Is Okay to Say "No"

Teens need to know they are in charge of their own bodies and they have a right to say "no" any time they don't feel comfortable. Counselors can empower teens to be aware of physical and sexual boundaries and to be able to enforce boundaries for their bodies. Teens need to also know that they don't owe their boyfriends or girlfriends sexual access to their bodies. They have a right to say "no" to their boyfriends or girlfriends. Healthy relationships for teens do not demand that teens be sexually active.

Counselors can also help teens place sexuality in the context of building a relationship. Frequently, teens believe intercourse establishes a relationship, rather than viewing sexuality as a component of a relationship. Counselors can assist teens in recognizing sexuality as one part of a relationship by helping teens develop criteria for engaging in sex. When counselors ask teens their criteria for engaging in sexual activities, the students may initially list statements like "A guy asks me" or "A girl says she likes me." Students can be encouraged to develop more selective criteria for engaging in sexual activities. The following questions provide some initial ideas for teens to consider.

1. Do I like this person?
2. How long have I known this person?
3. Do I trust this person?

4. Does this person care about me or is he or she faking it?
5. Is this person being nice to me because he or she wants me to have sex?
6. Do I feel pressured into having sex?
7. Am I choosing to have sex to be liked?

Summary

Counselors who understand adolescent development and how it affects teen decisions about sexuality can help teens cope with their changing bodies and their growing interest in sexuality. Counselors can accept teen concerns about sexual development, help teens recognize normal adolescent sexual issues, and develop skills to make decisions about their own sexuality.

3

You Are Not Immune: Pregnancy and Sexually Transmitted Diseases

If you are reading this chapter, we do not need to convince you that there is a growing problem with teenage pregnancy and sexually transmitted diseases (STDs). You can probably quote the statistics for us. You know that pregnancy and sexually transmitted diseases affect teens daily, but most teens do not believe that they will have to deal with these realities of being sexually active. You are no doubt familiar with statements like the following:

"I didn't plan for it to happen."

"I didn't know I could get pregnant the first time."

"It won't happen to me."

"It might happen to someone else, but I'm different."

"My boyfriend told me I wouldn't get pregnant."

"I only had sex with nice girls."

In contrast to teens who unwillingly or unintentionally become pregnant, there are teenagers who make an intentional choice to be sexually active and, in some cases, want to get pregnant and be a teenage parent. What can you do to educate students about pregnancy and STDs? What can you do to encourage parents to discuss sexual issues with their teens? What can you do to help teens make more responsible decisions? In this chapter, we will supply a number of sample lesson plans and activities for you to use in working with adolescents, parents, teachers, and community members.

Knowing What You Need to Know

The first step in providing effective interventions for sexually active teens is being knowledgeable about STDs and contraceptive methods. Counselors need to know that the following behaviors can help prevent STDs:

- Being selective when choosing a sex partner
- Limiting the number of sex partners
- Paying attention to warning signs of STDs
- Having regular physicals at a health clinic or a doctor's office
- Using latex or polyurethane condoms
- Practicing outercourse
- Having regular STD testing conducted
- Realizing that no one is immune from STDs

In addition, counselors should have a general knowledge of symptoms and methods of treatment for some of the most prevalent STDs. Table 3.1 provides an overview of STDs.

Although medical professionals will generally assist teens in making decisions concerning methods of contraception, counselors still need to be familiar with methods of contraception and their effectiveness in preventing pregnancies and STDs. Counselors should also have basic information concerning the advantages and disadvantages of different contraceptive methods. Table 3.2 provides an overview of different types of contraception and the effectiveness, advantages, disadvantages, and costs of these methods.

Being familiar with general information concerning STDs and pregnancy is the foundation for providing effective prevention and intervention for teens. Counselors who invest the time to learn about STDs and methods of contraception are prepared to develop counseling skills and prevention programs that will positively impact adolescents.

Seeing It Through Their Eyes

If you are going to build relationships with teens and help them develop skills to make responsible decisions about sexual issues, you have to see the world as they see it and hear the words the way they hear them. Teens do not perceive the world the way adults do, and as a result, they do not think the way adults do. In the movie *Dead Poets Society*, Mr. Keating, a teacher, stands on top of his desk and proclaims that he stands on top of his desk to remind himself that we must constantly look at things in a different way. He says the world looks different from the top of the desk because you are looking at things in a different way. As counselors, we must recognize that teens are seeing the world from a different perspective. If we are going to be effective, we are going to have to climb up on top of the desk to see the world from an adolescent's perspective. In the following section, we will present three different perspectives teens take about dealing with pregnancy and STDs.

text continues on page 41

TABLE 3.1 Overview of Sexually Transmitted Diseases (STDs)

STD	Symptom	Diagnosis	Treatment	Prevention
Chlamydia	75% of women and 25% of men have no symptoms. Women experience bleeding, abdominal pain, and vaginal discharge; usually occurs within a month. In men, symptoms include discharge, burning, and itching in the penis area; usually occurs within 3–5 days.	Lab exam	Antibiotics (usually Doxycycline or Azithromycin)	Condoms
Crabs	Intense itching	Direct observation	Nonprescription drugs or prescription lotion	Condoms
Genital herpes	Skin inflamed with red bumps and blisters. Pain occurs during urination.	Lab exam	Ointment and prescription (Acyclovir). Usually no cure.	Condoms help but are not totally effective.
Genital warts	No symptoms. Warts appear in genital area either as bumpy or flat.	Direct observation	Removal of wart by liquid medication or burning. Usually no cure.	Condoms help but are ineffective if condoms do not cover warts.

	Symptoms	Test	Treatment	Prevention
Gonorrhea (Clap)	Purulent penile discharge in men and urethritis or cervicitis in women. Incubation period is 2-8 days; asymptomatic carriers occur in both men and women, although more common in women.	Lab test (culture)	Antibiotics	Condoms
Hepatitis B	Many have no symptoms. Some have dark urine, jaundice, and/or symptoms like a stomach virus.	Lab test (blood test)	There is no cure. The only treatment is rest combined with a high-protein and high-carbohydrate diet.	Condoms, and vaccination prior to the infection.
HIV/AIDS	Being tired, losing weight, and having permanent diarrhea. Swollen glands are very prevalent.	Lab test (blood test)	There is no cure. Some prescriptions lengthen survival.	Condoms. Avoid sharing needles (drugs).
Syphilis	Occurs as painless genital ulcers in primary stage. Occurs as rash and/or lymph node enlargement in secondary stage. Often in late stage, no symptoms but may occur with signs of vascular and neurological damage.	Lab exam (fluid)	Penicillin or Doxycycline	Condoms and spermicides

Source: Adapted from Leukefeld & Haverkos (1993).

TABLE 3.2 Methods of Contraception

Method	Effectiveness	Advantages	Disadvantages	Cost
Abstinence: You and your partner do not engage in vaginal intercourse.	Pregnancy: 100% STDs: 100%	No medical side effects. Women who postpone vaginal intercourse until their 20s are less likely to suffer from STDs, infertility, and cancer of the cervix.	Difficult to abstain from intercourse for long periods of time. People forget to protect themselves when they stop abstaining.	None
Outercourse: You enjoy sex play without vaginal intercourse, which keeps sperm from joining egg.	Pregnancy: Nearly 100% STDs: Nearly 100%	No medical side effects. May prolong sex play and enhance orgasm. Can be satisfying without the risks of sexual intercourse.	May be difficult for people to abstain from vaginal intercourse for long periods of time.	None
Norplant: A physician will put six small capsules under the skin of your upper arm. These release hormones preventing the release of an egg and thicken cervical mucus to keep sperm from joining egg.	Pregnancy: 99.96% STDs: Not effective	Protects against pregnancy for 5 years. No daily pill. Nothing to put in place before intercourse.	Irregular, late, absent periods. Discomforts including: headaches, nausea, depression, nervousness, dizziness, and weight gain. Medical procedure needed for insertion and removal.	Exam/insertion: $500-$600 Removal: $100-$200

Method	Effectiveness	Benefits	Side Effects/Risks	Cost
Depo-Provera: A shot in your arm or buttock every 12 weeks. Prevents the release of an egg, thickens cervical mucus to keep sperm from joining egg, and prevents fertilized egg from implanting in uterus.	Pregnancy: 99.7% STDs: Not effective	Protects against pregnancy for 12 weeks. No daily pill. Nothing to put in place before intercourse. Protects against cancer of the uterus and iron deficiency anemia.	Irregular, late, and absent periods. Discomforts including: weight gain, headaches, depression, and abdominal pain. Side effects cannot be reversed until medication wears off (up to 12 weeks).	Injection: $30-$75 Exam: $35-$125
The Pill: A pill taken once a day. The pills contain hormones that prevent the release of an egg, thicken cervical mucus to keep sperm from joining egg, and prevent fertilized egg from implanting in uterus.	Pregnancy: 97%-99.9% STDs: Not effective	Nothing to put in place before intercourse. More regular periods. Less menstrual cramping, acne, iron deficiency anemia, premenstrual tension. Protects against ovarian and endometrial cancers, pelvic inflammatory disease, and noncancerous breast tumors.	Must be taken daily. Rare health risks including blood clots, heart attack, and stroke. Discomforts including temporary irregular bleeding, depression, and nausea.	Monthly pills: $15-$25 Exam: $35-$125
Condom: A sheath that covers the penis before intercourse to keep sperm from joining egg.	Pregnancy: 88%-98% STDs: Latex condoms are effective.	Inexpensive and easy to buy. Can help relieve premature ejaculation. Can be used with other methods of birth control.	Allergies to latex or spermicide. Decreased sensation. Breakage.	$.25-$2.50

39

TABLE 3.2 Continued

Method	Effectiveness	Advantages	Disadvantages	Cost
Diaphragm/Cervical cap: A physician fits you with a shallow latex cup (diaphragm) or a thimble-shaped latex cup (cervical cap). The diaphragm or cap can be coated with spermicide and put in your vagina to keep sperm from joining the egg.	Pregnancy: 64%-94% STDs: Not effective.	No medical side effects. Inexpensive.	Can be messy. Allergies to latex or spermicide. Cannot use during vaginal bleeding or infection.	Diaphragm/Cap: $13-$25 Exam: $50-$125
Vaginal Pouch/Spermicides: Spermicides that immobilize sperm include contraceptive foam, cream, jelly, film, or suppository. Both are inserted into vagina shortly before intercourse.	Pregnancy: 72%-97% STDs: Pouch provides some protection.	Easy to buy. Erection unnecessary to keep pouch in place.	Can be messy. Allergies and may irritate vagina or penis. Difficulty inserting pouch. Outer ring of pouch may slip into the vagina during intercourse.	$2.50-$18.00

SOURCE: Adapted from Planned Parenthood, 1997.

Don't Think About It at All

Many students engage in sexual activity without giving consideration to a variety of physical, emotional, and relational consequences. Six weeks ago, Janet had an argument with her parents. After the argument, she went to a party with her boyfriend, Jeff. At the party, she wanted to forget about arguing with her parents and have fun. She drank a lot that night. The next day, she couldn't remember what she did the night before. She remembered having sex with someone and hoped it was with Jeff. Janet had an upset stomach for a couple of days and went to see her doctor. Her worst fear was realized. She came to your office and told you that she was pregnant. You knew Janet took health and biology classes that discussed contraceptives. She knew how to prevent a pregnancy, but she didn't.

Janet typifies a group of teens who may not think about pregnancy or STDs at all. When teens use drugs or alcohol, their ability to consider the consequences of their actions is impaired. Janet's knowledge about contraception and even strong values about sexuality did not prevent her from getting pregnant. In some cases, teens are not under the influence of drugs or alcohol. They are sexually aroused and act impulsively without thinking about the potential consequences of pregnancy and STDs. One student said, "It's not like I try to think about sex all the time. I can be walking down the halls at school and all of a sudden my body does this. It's not like our bodies aren't intended to have sex."

Regardless of whether teens are under the influence of drugs or alcohol or are acting impulsively, the reality is that they often do not think about the consequences of their sexual activities and are at risk for STDs and/or pregnancy. Effective prevention programs will recognize that teens may not think about the consequences of sexual activities and will be designed to assist students in anticipating and evaluating the consequences of being sexually active.

Don't Think It Can Happen to Me

A second perspective students take is the belief that they will not get pregnant or contract an STD because normal consequences do not apply to them. When Danny was first sexually active, he initially engaged in sexual intercourse only with his girlfriend, but once they broke up, he had sex with several other partners. When Danny started having a burning sensation when he urinated, he went to the school health clinic. Danny was stunned when he was told that a lab test confirmed he had chlamydia. The nurse explained to Danny that chlamydia was an STD and referred Danny to a counselor.

"I can't believe this happened to me. I was always careful about sex. I never thought this could happen to me," says Danny. Danny had not really listened in health class when information about STDs was presented because he did not think he could catch an STD. Danny's situation is characteristic of teens who believe pregnancies and STDs cannot happen to them. This "it won't happen to me" attitude is reflective of normal adolescent development. Teens believe that normal consequences do not apply to them. Adolescents are more concerned with immediate effects of behaviors than long-term effects of behaviors.

Effective intervention programs will recognize students may have the perspective that normal consequences do not apply to them. In response to this perspective, intervention programs will move beyond presenting statistics and information and will help teens personalize the possibility of getting pregnant or contracting an STD.

Want It to Happen to Me

The third perspective teens take is that they want to get someone pregnant or get pregnant themselves. Susan's parents divorced 10 years ago, and Susan's mom remarried and started a second family. Susan felt left out at home and wanted to feel loved. She dated to fill the void in her life, a void that she experienced following her parents' divorce. When Susan and Ted began having intercourse, Susan took birth control pills. Gradually, she quit taking the pills because she believed that having a baby would bring Ted closer to her. When Susan thought about getting pregnant, she pictured herself getting married to Ted and both of them raising their baby together. Susan discovered she was pregnant and was stunned by Ted's reaction to the pregnancy. He suggested she get an abortion because a pregnancy could "mess up" their lives. Susan talked to a counselor because she didn't know what to do. She said, "I thought having a baby would make Ted love me more."

Susan is representative of a group of teenagers who may want to get pregnant because of the perceived benefits of pregnancy. In some cases, pregnancy may have a benefit for the teenager, but in most cases, the teenager has a misperception concerning the benefits of pregnancy. As you talk with teens who want to get pregnant, you need to assess the reasons why a teenager wants to get pregnant. Following is a list of some of the perceived benefits of pregnancy.

1. *Power.* Teens perceive that pregnancy will enhance their power to make choices in their lives by giving them "adult" status. Realistically, when teenagers become parents, they typically emancipate and gain legal status as adults.

2. *Control.* Teens may use pregnancy to control other people. The pregnant adolescent may use the pregnancy to force a boyfriend to marry her or to compel her parents to comply with her wishes or desires.

3. *Intimacy.* Teens equate sex with intimacy. Instead of developing intimacy and then becoming sexually active, teenagers may have the misperception that sexual involvement creates emotional intimacy. Teens believe having a baby will create more intimacy with their sexual partner. Likewise, adolescent females feel their child will help meet their needs for intimacy.

4. *Escape.* Teens view pregnancy as an avenue of escape. Adolescents who are experiencing difficulties at home or want to move out of their parents' homes may believe getting pregnant will allow them to move into another household or to establish a household of their own. Pregnancy may also allow teenagers to escape the expectations others have for them concerning achievement and status.

5. *Rebellion.* Pregnancy is also a means of rebelling against parental authority. If teenagers know their parents dislike their sexual

partners, or are opposed to them being sexually active or becoming pregnant, a pregnancy is the ultimate "in your face" act for a teenager.

6. *Purpose.* Pregnancy can be an avenue, especially for females, to form a relationship with someone that will love them and give them a sense of purpose in life.

7. *Procreation.* Teens may see pregnancy as a way to pass on part of themselves to the next generation. The infant becomes a symbol of making a lasting legacy or contribution.

Part of Who I Am

In considering the reasons why teenagers get pregnant, cultural issues should be considered. Culture is more than race. Ethnicity, nationality, language, religion, age, sex, and socioeconomic status are all elements of culture. A cultural group may view pregnancy and/or parenthood as a rite of passage into adulthood and may not view teenage pregnancy as a negative situation.

The school counselor saw Rogelio in the hall and said, "Hey Rogelio, how are you doin'?"

"Great, man. Things are really goin' great."

"Sounds like some good things are happenin'."

"My girlfriend's going to have a baby. It's my baby. I'm a man."

"Your girlfriend's pregnant?"

"Yeah, ain't it great! I'm a player."

Rogelio's dialogue reflects changing cultural norms. Rogelio is proud that he has gotten his girlfriend pregnant because he believes it proves his masculinity. Rogelio's perspective on fathering children is not limited to teens. Professional athletes model this behavior for teens. Larry Johnson, a professional basketball player, is supporting five children by four different women. LaTrell Sprewell, another professional basketball player, had three children by three different women before he was 21 years old. These men, as well as other professional athletes, serve as models for teens. What they model for teens is an emphasis on instant gratification with no thought of how today's pleasure may impact tomorrow's options or obligations.

Rogelio's conversation is reflective of a group of teens who may actually even try to get more than one girl pregnant at a time to establish adult status.

In contrast to the description of Rogelio, the counselor should consider how a culture may view pregnancy negatively and how pregnancy and/or teen parenthood could result in being ostracized from one's cultural group. Counselors should explore questions with teenagers such as the following:

- How does your cultural group view pregnancy outside of marriage?
- What would a teenager gain in your culture if he or she was a parent?
- What would a teenager lose in your culture if he or she was a parent?
- What would a teenager gain by getting married in your culture?
- What resources would be available to teenage parents in your culture?

Planning Effective Prevention Programs

Prevention programs in schools, if they exist, predominantly focus on sex education. Traditionally, these programs emphasize the biological aspects of sex and stress abstinence. Although abstinence may be the only model that is 100% effective in preventing pregnancy and STDs, the reality is that a growing number of adolescents become sexually active at younger ages. These programs have emphasized a banking model where information is deposited, but little else is done to promote responsible decision making about sexual issues. Students may have biological information, but they don't connect that information with what happens when they are making out in a car or in someone's bedroom. These programs have failed to engage students in interacting with each other and adults. Through this type of interaction, students learn to process information in a personal way, making it relevant to how they make decisions. Although an understanding of anatomy and physiology is necessary, teens also need to know about emotional and physical consequences of sexual activity. Effective prevention and intervention programs targeting sexual behavior must address emotional and physical consequences by being

- *Persistent:* Effective preventive programs have a repeated, consistent message concerning sexual behavior and its consequences with an emphasis on making responsible decisions. Teenagers hear about sexuality issues frequently and repeatedly rather than once a year in a health or biology class.
- *Comprehensive:* Effective prevention programs begin in elementary school and continue throughout the educational experience. In addition, effective programs involve school administrators, teachers, health care professionals, community members, and parents.
- *Supportive:* Effective prevention programs stress the importance of supportive adult relationships. Teenagers are struggling to develop their own identity and values and need supportive adults who will encourage them to develop their decision-making skills and a sense of self-competency. Providing emotional support can deter teenagers from seeking intimacy in sexual relationships.
- *Competency-based:* Effective prevention programs help teenagers develop competencies to assist in making decisions about their own sexuality. Competency enhancement can emphasize social skills training, decision making, and problem-solving skills.

Getting Students Involved

Classroom guidance activities. Perhaps one of the easiest ways to educate students about the risks of pregnancy and STDs is through classroom guidance activities. Different types of messages are effective in working with adolescents at different ages. The physical aspects of sexual activity are more meaningful for 12-year-olds, while social and psychological concerns increase in importance with age. Regardless of the age of the students, students should realize that it is not who they are, but what they do that places them at risk.

Classroom guidance activities emphasizing lectures or a myth-versus-fact approach are not effective. For classroom guidance activities to be effective, they must require that adolescents actively participate. Counselors can encourage active participation using questionnaires, games, and role-playing. In addition, using multimedia presentations such as videos or contemporary music is even more effective. Sample outlines of classroom guidance activities are provided on the following pages. These outlines are intended to be examples and must be adapted to various needs, cultures, and ages. Hopefully, they will get you thinking about other things you can do in your own unique setting.

Classroom Guidance Activity Sample Outline:
Know Your Contraceptives

At the beginning of this activity, the counselor should divide participants into five groups. A large piece of poster board is divided into columns with headings listing contraceptive methods. The first group of participants is given 1 minute to match note cards containing descriptions of contraceptive methods with the methods' names on the poster board. When time expires, the group scores points based on the number of correct answers. The presenter moves the descriptions to the correct column on the poster board if necessary. Participants in the other groups are given a set of note cards to match to names of contraceptive methods. The other groups of note cards cover effectiveness, advantages, disadvantages, and costs of contraceptive methods. Information about contraceptive methods is found in Table 3.1. (The same activity can be used for information about STDs found in Table 3.2.) When students complete the activity, the counselor discusses which contraceptive methods are *not* recommended for teens based on the following information (Planned Parenthood, 1997):

1. *Sterilization.* An individual has an operation to keep sperm from joining the egg. Sterilization is not recommended for teens because

it is intended to be permanent and is not appropriate for anyone who may want to have a child in the future.

2. *IUD (Intrauterine device).* A physician puts a small plastic device in the uterus. The IUD contains copper or hormones that keep sperm from joining the egg or preventing the fertilized egg from implanting in the uterus. An IUD is not recommended for teens because a young woman's uterus may be too small to hold an IUD. In addition, IUD users who contract certain STDs may develop pelvic inflammatory disease and be unable to have children.

3. *Withdrawal.* The man withdraws his penis from the vagina before he ejaculates to keep sperm from joining the egg. The withdrawal method is not recommended for teens because

- Some men lack the experience and self-control to pull out in time
- Some men say they will pull out but get carried away and don't
- Some men cannot tell when they are going to ejaculate
- Before ejaculation, almost all penises leak fluid that can cause pregnancy

4. *Periodic abstinence.* A medical professional teaches a female how to chart her menstrual cycle and detect certain physical signs to help predict 9 or more days during the menstrual cycle when she is more likely to get pregnant. Periodic abstinence is not recommended for teens because this method works best for adult women with very regular periods. Furthermore, teenage sexual partners may not wish to cooperate in using this method.

Classroom Guidance Activity Sample Outline:
Myths Concerning Contraception

The counselor selects participants to portray teen characters who are sexually active but are not using contraception. The counselor should give the teens portraying the characters a note card outlining why the character is not using contraception. Participants question the teen characters to determine why they are not using contraception. The teen character answers the questions based on the reason on the note card. Some reasons why teenagers might not use contraception include the following:

"I'll get fat if I start taking the pill."

"If I use a condom, it will interrupt the flow of things."

"I can't get pregnant the first time I have sex."

"My boyfriend told me not to worry about getting pregnant."

As each role-play concludes, the counselor encourages participants to explore why teens believe they do not need to use contraception. The role-plays are used as a catalyst to explore participants' perceptions.

Student support groups. Adolescents are trying to develop an identity away from their families for the first time and need supportive peer relationships. Support groups can provide students with a venue for discussing sexuality issues in a nonthreatening manner, particularly if older adolescents can be trained to be facilitators for the group. Teenagers are more likely to listen to peers rather than adults. A support group gives students a chance to explore their own values about sexuality and their own approaches to intimacy with their peers.

Peer mentoring. Another way to involve teenagers with their peers in positive relationships is through the development of a peer mentoring program. A peer mentoring program allows students to improve decision-making skills and learn appropriate social skills in a nonthreatening way with a peer role model. Peer mentors can dispel some myths teenagers have about sexuality.

Resource centers. One of the easiest and most effective ways to provide information for teenagers about sexuality is to develop a resource center. The resource center needs to be easily accessible and should provide students with handouts, pamphlets, books, and videos that address teenage concerns and decisions about sexuality. Handouts and pamphlets should be made available for students to take with them as a permanent resource. In contrast, students check out or borrow videos or books (see Resources at the end of this book for a list of available resources).

Getting Parents Involved

Parent-child communication workshops. The quality of the relationship between parents and adolescents is a major factor in whether teens will talk with their parents about sexual issues. The school counselor can provide opportunities for parents and teens to develop effective communication patterns before problems exist. Then, if problems arise, the foundation for effective communication already exists. The emphasis in the workshops should be to help parents identify ways to communicate their family values and boundaries. The workshops should help parents learn to use "I" messages in discussing conflicts and to use nonthreatening language to communicate boundaries. In addition, the workshop should emphasize the importance of communication about sexual issues. The workshops should practice strategies that build skills and involve role-plays. A sample outline for a communication workshop for parents follows.

> *Communication Workshop Sample Outline:*
> *How Do I Talk About Sexual Stuff?*

Introduction. The counselor should introduce himself or herself and explain the purpose of the workshop is to improve communication skills for discussing sexual issues. The counselor should encourage participants to express their opinions and feelings. Likewise, the participants should be encouraged to listen to other participants and accept other participants' feelings without being critical or judgmental.

Activity: Telephone call (adapted from MacBeth & Fine, 1995). The counselor instructs participants to work in pairs. Each participant sits back-to-back with his or her partner. One participant is the caller, and the other is the receiver. The caller gets a problem written on a card, but the problem is not revealed to the receiver. The problem could be

- You are being pressured by a boyfriend or girlfriend to have sex
- You are 16 and pregnant
- You are sexually active and want information about contraceptives
- You are diagnosed with an STD
- You are a victim of date rape
- A peer is sexually harassing you

The caller starts talking, but does not immediately reveal the problem. The caller finds it difficult to discuss the problem and needs to be encouraged by the receiver. The caller may hint at the problem, talk about it indirectly, or talk about something unrelated. The receiver encourages the caller to discuss the problem and make decisions. At the end of the role-play, the caller gives feedback to the listener before reversing roles for a different role-play. At the end of the activity, all participants discuss what they learned from the experience and how they felt in both roles.

Activity: Finding ways to talk. To introduce the activity, the counselor explains that sexual issues can be discussed more effectively in many brief interactions rather than in one long "sex talk." Hypothetical situations or media presentations provide a nonthreatening way to discuss sexuality with teens.

Role-Play Number 1

The counselor selects participants to portray a teenager and a parent in a role-play. The parent and teenager have been watching a sitcom on television. A character in the sitcom is deciding if he or she wants to be sexually active. The parent begins the role-play with the following statement: "That character had some difficult choices to make. What would you have done in that situation?"

percent effective in preventing other sexually transmitted diseases, and it appears that they are similarly effective in preventing HIV transmission. But condoms are not foolproof.

Here we come to the delicate part. I need to tell you how to use a condom, much as I don't want to. First, a word of caution—don't use petroleum products or jellies (like Vaseline) with condoms. The latex breaks down with petroleum jellies and the virus is able to pass through the condom. A condom comes packed in a sealed pouch, and it's rolled up like the base of a balloon. Make sure the package is sealed and new because condoms deteriorate when they get old. When they are old, they can break apart. That's a disaster because sperm and the virus will move through the latex.

When the condom is put on, it's rolled over the male's erect penis. Space must be left at the end—a reservoir at the tip of the condom to catch the sperm. The end is pinched and pulled before rolling it on. After sex, the condom must be held at the base of the penis when it is removed so the sperm remains in the condom. You got it?

Whew! That's enough for now. I'm glad I told you. I'm a little scared in the back of my mind that you'll use this information to have sexual experiences. It's probably a baseless fear. I think I know better than that and really do feel better that you have this information. If you have any questions, your mom and dad are here for you. Never forget that we love you and wish only that you live as well and wisely as you can.

Love, Dad

Conclusion. The counselor should review the concepts learned during the workshop. The counselor should have participants write one thing on a note card that they can change to improve communication with their teenager.

Parent support groups. The purpose of a parent support group is to provide information and support to parents of adolescents. Topics for a support group can include communicating with your teen, being a trustworthy parent, keeping secrets, understanding teen sexuality, and preventing teen pregnancy. Parent support groups provide an opportunity for parents to discuss issues such as boundary setting and ways to set limits for dating and socializing with peers.

Parent education presentations. Presentations for parents emphasize the importance of communicating values, nurturing healthy adolescent sexuality, understanding consequences of teenage pregnancy, and preventing STDs. The following outlines are provided to give some ideas for presentations.

Parent Presentation Sample Outline:
What I Want My Child to Know About Sex

Introduction. The counselor should introduce himself or herself and explain that the purpose of the presentation is to identify which values the participants want to communicate to their teenagers about sexual issues. The counselor should encourage participants to express their opinions and feelings openly, while listening to other participants without being critical or judgmental.

Activity: When I was a teenager. The counselor explains to participants that adolescence is a unique time when teenagers experience changes in the way they think and the way their bodies react. Parents can better understand these changes if they reflect on their own experiences during adolescence. The counselor should have participants complete a handout with the following items.

When I was a teenager . . . .

What scared me most about dating was _____ .

What I disliked most about my body was _____ .

What scared me most about sex was _____ .

What my parents communicated about sex was _____ .

What I enjoyed most about dating was _____ .

My first date was _____ .

My first kiss was _____ .

The person I talked to about sex was _____ .

Once participants complete the handout, they should discuss in pairs their answers on the worksheet. The counselor should then place participants in groups of six and have them list themes that were common in their answers. Participants share themes with the entire group at the conclusion of the activity.

Activity: What a teenager needs to know. A large sheet of paper should be divided into columns. The columns are identified as the following: dating, contraception, sexually transmitted diseases, and sexual activity. Participants share words or short phrases describing what they would like their teens to know about each of these sexual issues. Participants chart those words or phrases on the paper. Participants do not debate or question why words or phrases are chosen. After all the participants have charted their ideas, participants can ask each other questions about the chart. The presenter should remind participants to avoid critical or judgmental remarks. Following the discussion, participants should write a brief statement about what they want their children to know about each of these sexual issues.

Conclusion. At the end of the presentation, the counselor gives participants strips of poster board and asks them to write down one thing they learned from the presentation.

Getting the Community Involved

Field trips. One of the easiest and most effective ways to involve the community is through school field trips to local agencies that provide services for teens who are sexually active or who are pregnant. Field trips should be planned to health clinics, drug abuse centers, treatment centers, and community agencies that provide services for teenage parents.

Adult mentoring programs. Adult mentoring programs can use community members to serve as role models for students and to assist students in developing their career goals. Students who have long-term goals for themselves are less likely to engage in risky behaviors. Role models can also help alter teenagers' misconceptions about sexuality and help inoculate them against media influences that promote sexual risk taking.

Community service programs. Involving adolescents in community service programs helps them build self-esteem and feel that they have a purpose in the community. Community service projects like Habitat for Humanity and local food banks are always looking for volunteers. Helping adolescents become involved in these community service projects can help them feel connected to the community and help them begin to build their own identity as citizens in the community.

Oh No! It's Happened to Me

When preventive interventions have not been successful, you may have to deal with teenagers who are pregnant or who have STDs. Before providing services for teens who are pregnant or who have STDs, you need to be aware of local school policies and state laws that apply to teenage pregnancy and other teenage sexuality issues. You also need to be aware of community agencies that provide services for teenagers who are pregnant or who have STDs. Community agencies will probably be better equipped to provide long-term counseling services for these teenagers than you are as a school counselor. Your role will probably involve making an initial assessment and then referring teens to the appropriate community resources. The following five-step model should assist you in these tasks.

1. Assess the client's immediate needs.
2. Refer the client for medical care.
3. Decide whom to notify.

4. Identify supportive relationships.
5. Consider long-term options.

This model will be used in two case studies to demonstrate how to intervene with a pregnant teenager and a teenager who has a STD.

Pregnancy

Sam and Lupe are both sophomores at Central High. Sam plays football and hopes to get an athletic scholarship for college. Lupe is the editor of the school paper and an honor student who hopes to earn an academic scholarship for college. Lupe and Sam dated on several occasions, but Lupe was startled last month when she discovered that she was pregnant. Lupe was confused about what to do. She was scared to discuss the situation with her parents, so she scheduled an appointment to visit with the school counselor. The counselor took the following steps to assist Lupe.

1. *Assess the client's immediate needs.* Lupe initially voiced several concerns about her health and the baby's health. The counselor gave her some information about prenatal development. In addition, Lupe was confused about her options and was scared to tell her parents and boyfriend. The counselor helped Lupe realize that refusing to address the pregnancy was not going to improve the situation. The counselor also stressed to Lupe that a pregnancy would alter her life if she decided to parent the child, but she could still make choices to provide options for herself and her child.

2. *Refer the client for medical care.* Because of her religious beliefs, Lupe did not want to consider the option of abortion. Her school counselor was aware of local services available to pregnant teenagers and referred her to a local health care clinic for prenatal care.

3. *Decide whom to notify.* Before discussing whom to notify, the counselor needs to be aware of state laws as well as school policies involving teen pregnancy. In some states, Lupe's parents might need to be notified, whereas in other states Lupe could decide whether to tell her parents. Lupe initially hesitated to discuss the

situation with Sam, but felt that she needed to let him know about the situation. Sam agreed to come with Lupe to meet with the school counselor. Sam and Lupe both agreed that marriage was not an option for them because they had only a casual dating relationship. However, Sam was willing to help provide emotional support and financial support for the baby.

Lupe had great difficulty deciding whether to tell her parents. The school counselor was careful to allow Lupe to make the decision. After three counseling sessions, Lupe acknowledged that her parents would have to be told if she was going to continue to live with them. Lupe's parents were initially upset, but were able to help Lupe consider long-term responsibilities.

4. *Identify supportive relationships.* Although Sam and Lupe's parents were willing to be supportive, she also needed the support of her peers. Like other pregnant and parenting adolescents, Lupe felt rejected by her peers, who were uncomfortable around her because she was pregnant. She found that because few of her "old" friends understood her concerns about her pregnancy, they were unwilling to support her. Lupe felt isolated from her peers after they learned that she was pregnant. The school counselor referred her to a local community agency that conducted support groups for pregnant teenagers and teenage parents. Lupe found that the relationships she developed in the support groups helped fill the void left by the departure of her other friends.

5. *Consider long-term options.* The school counselor assisted Lupe in making plans about her educational future and career goals. Lupe decided to attend school at an alternative educational campus. In the alternative educational program, Lupe not only attended academic-skills classes, but also attended parenting-skills classes. In addition to academic training, medical and nutritional needs were discussed and provided. Perhaps one of the greatest advantages of the program was that child-care services were provided on-site at the school where Lupe attended classes.

In addition to assistance with educational goals, Lupe also needed financial assistance and access to long-term medical care. The school counselor referred Lupe to a local social service agency that helped her complete applications for the Special Supplemental Food Program for Women, Infants, and Children (WIC). WIC provides assistance with food for eligible pregnant and lactating women and children less than 5 years old. Lupe also qualified for assistance from Aid to Families with Dependent Children (AFDC) and Medicaid.

Sexually Transmitted Diseases

Susan was just diagnosed with HIV. For 2 years, she dated the manager of the restaurant where she worked. At first, they smoked pot, and then later they advanced to IV drug use. Their days and evenings were often spent sharing needles with other drug users. About 5 months ago, Susan experienced flu-like symptoms that would not go away. As the days progressed, Susan felt listless. It was as if getting out of bed was getting more difficult by the day. Finally, Susan decided to see her doctor who gave her a prescription. Although she took the prescription as directed, she didn't feel any better and went back to see her doctor again. Her doctor did a thorough exam including lab tests and informed Susan that she was HIV-positive. Susan was stunned by the diagnosis and went to talk with her school counselor.

1. *Assess the client's immediate needs.* Susan told her counselor that she was frightened. She believed the diagnosis of being HIV-positive was a death sentence. The counselor helped Susan recognize that she could live an active life for years with the HIV infection. In addition, Susan was concerned that when her family and friends realized she was HIV-positive they would refuse to interact with her. The counselor emphasized the importance of educating people about how HIV infection is not transmitted through casual contact. HIV infection is only transmitted through bodily fluids like blood, mucus, and semen.

2. *Refer the client for medical care.* The counselor did not have to refer Susan for medical care because Susan had already contacted her doctor.

3. *Decide whom to notify.* Susan had great difficulty deciding whom to tell that she was HIV-positive. Although she knew her parents would be devastated, she felt that she needed their support and a chance to talk with them about her fears and concerns. When Susan told her parents, they were quite distraught initially, but then contacted the local AIDS social service agency to obtain information about HIV and AIDS. Susan told her boyfriend, and he tested positive for the HIV virus. When he found out that he was HIV-positive, he blamed Susan and severed his relationship with her.

4. *Identify supportive relationships.* In addition to the support of her parents, Susan needed support from her peers. The school counselor referred Susan to the local AIDS community agency. Susan became involved in a support group facilitated by the agency and developed relationships with several other teenagers who were HIV positive.

5. *Consider long-term options.* Because Susan's health was not significantly impaired, she attended school on a regular basis and continued her involvement in extracurricular activities.

Summary

The foundation for effective intervention and prevention is being knowledgeable about STDs, pregnancy, and contraceptive options. In addition, school counselors need to consider how developmental and family issues affect the way teens make decisions about being sexually active. In addition, counselors who develop effective prevention programs integrate knowledge about adolescent development with an outreach to students, parents, and community members. With a systematic approach to prevention, counselors can help teens avoid STDs and pregnancy. However, no approach to prevention is going to be 100% effective. Counselors will still need to help teens cope with STDs and pregnancy and provide appropriate support and services to meet their needs.

Certainly, no counseling program can eliminate all STDs and pregnancy. Rather than evaluating the effectiveness of a program in terms of rates of STDs and pregnancies, success can be measured in terms of the students' willingness to discuss the issues of STDs and pregnancy and the counselor's willingness to dialogue openly with students about the possible negative outcomes of choosing to be sexually active.

4

This Isn't Supposed to Happen: Dealing With Sexual Violence

A student tells you that she thinks her best friend has been raped. A teacher asks you to talk with a student because the teacher suspects sexual abuse. A coach suspects another coach may be sexually involved with a student. Dealing with issues of sexual abuse, incest, and rape may be the most overwhelming tasks a school counselor faces. While teenagers integrating sexuality into their self-concept is part of the normal cycle of human development, sexual violence is not part of the normal developmental sequence. Sexual violence presents a challenging situation for counselors. Counselors may frequently be called on to provide crisis intervention, to make immediate decisions involving social service agencies and/or the police, and to testify in court. This chapter is written to help you make the appropriate decisions and provide effective intervention for students with sexual violence issues.

What Should I Look For?

Sheila, a junior, was involved in a number of disciplinary issues during the school year. She was rude and disrespectful in talking with her teachers and, at times, was defiant and refused to comply with her teachers' requests. In addition, she was sent home on several occasions to change her clothes because her skirts or shorts were "indecent." Her inappropriate behavior escalated as the school year progressed. Her grades dropped, and she cut classes. In the past month, she was referred to the assistant principal three times for fighting with another female student during the school day. On her third referral to the assistant principal, Sheila was told she would be referred to an alternative school program if she had another major disciplinary problem. The assistant principal noticed Sheila was an excellent student in junior high and was not referred for discipline problems at all until the current school year. The assistant principal decided to ask the school counselor to visit with Sheila and to provide assistance.

At first glance, Sheila's disciplinary problems do not seem related to a discussion of sexual abuse, but they are. Sheila's disciplinary problems could be indicative of sexual abuse, incest, or rape. Teenagers may manifest their anger and frustration by acting aggressively toward others or by refusing to comply with adult instructions. Disclosures of abuse may occur as a result of a teenager being punished for inappropriate behaviors—behaviors that may be unrecognized symptoms of sexual abuse or incest. The following description of symptoms of sexual violence can be used to help you identify students who may need assistance in dealing with sexual abuse or rape.

Somatic complaints. Sexually abused teenagers may complain of physical symptoms including stomachaches, headaches, vomiting, leg cramps, nausea, and itching or soreness in genital or rectal areas.

Promiscuous behaviors. Frequently, promiscuous behavior with peers and/or provocative behavior with adults may be indications of sexual abuse or incest. Teenagers who have experienced sexual abuse may demonstrate inappropriate sexual boundaries by touching others, wearing seductive clothing or demonstrating seductive postures, removing clothing in inappropriate situations, masturbating frequently or in public, and openly asking for sex. In some cases, sexual abuse may lead to teenagers' engaging in prostitution.

Delinquency. Teenagers who are sexually abused are likely to be initially referred to a school counselor for expressing their anger through misconduct. Delinquent behaviors may include using drugs and/or alcohol, running away, being truant, and acting aggressively toward others.

Compliance. Refusing to comply with adult instructions and acting overly compliant toward adult requests are two extremes of behavior that may indicate sexual abuse. Resisting authority, mistreating adults, and behaving poorly may reflect a refusal to comply with adult requests, whereas excessive concern about pleasing adults may signal that a student is overly compliant.

Attention problems. Short attention span, learning problems, and task-completion difficulties may be symptoms of sexual abuse. In addition, a sudden drop in school grades or performance in class may reflect that school has lost importance for the sexually abused teenager.

Depression. Teenagers who have experienced sexual abuse may exhibit symptoms of depression. These include listlessness, crying easily or frequently, changing eating or sleeping habits, being irritable, having low self-esteem, or attempting suicide.

Poor self-image. Indications of poor self-image that may be exhibited by sexually abused teenagers include poor hygiene, lack of concern about appearance, negative statements about self such as

"I'm dumb and ugly" or "I don't deserve to be loved," ideas that
they "deserve" punishment, and self-abusive behaviors.

Withdrawal. As a result of sexual abuse, teenagers may socially
withdraw and isolate themselves from others. In addition, they
may have poor peer relationships and difficulty relating to individuals their own age. Teenagers may be extremely secretive or
feel they are unique and different, so they have nothing in common with their peers. Withdrawal may be manifested in little
involvement in or an unwillingness to participate in social, physical, or recreational activities. In some cases, withdrawal may even
lead to the client's living in a fantasy world rather than acknowl-
edging reality.

Family issues. Family patterns of communication and interaction
may be especially indicative of incest. Sexual abuse or incest may
result in role reversals in families where children are protective of
parents or assume excessive household duties. Poor relationships
with one parent or excessive time spent alone with one parent may
indicate an incestuous relationship. Favoritism toward one child,
jealousy of a child's relationships outside the family, and jealousy
of a particular sibling may also indicate incest.

As the previous discussion indicates, Sheila's inappropriate behaviors could indicate that she experienced sexual abuse, incest, or
rape. She exhibited the following behaviors: violations of the dress
code, changes in her grades and truancy, a refusal to comply with
teachers' instructions, physical aggression, and difficulty in peer
relationships. Sheila did not exhibit all the behaviors that could be
related to sexual violence. However, a counselor should be looking
for a pattern of several of these behaviors—not necessarily all of
them—as an indication of sexual abuse, incest, or rape. These behaviors may be an indication of sexual violence, but Sheila's behaviors
may also be reflective of parental marital difficulties, a significant loss
in her life, or any number of other situations. If a student manifests
some of these symptoms or even most of these symptoms, the counselor cannot automatically *assume* the student has experienced sexual
violence, but the counselor should consider the possibility of sexual

abuse, incest, or rape and be willing to explore the possibility with the student.

How Do I Find Out?

Let's suppose that the school counselor has scheduled a time to visit with Sheila. How would the counselor approach a discussion of the possibility of sexual abuse with Sheila? The counselor would need to create a safe place for Sheila to disclose information regarding sexual violence. The physical environment needs to offer security from interruptions and distractions. The counselor needs to close the office door, close blinds or curtains, and prohibit interruptions from secretaries, teachers, and administrators. Similarly, the counselor needs to prevent telephone interruptions by turning off the ringer on the phone or by allowing an answering machine to pick up calls. Teenagers are not going to discuss a private issue when they fear someone may walk in on the middle of the conversation. In addition, the office needs to be a welcoming place, preferably with comfortable chairs and posters or decorations that are appropriate for teenagers.

Once you have established a safe place for teenagers to disclose, you next need to develop counseling skills that will promote disclosure. Let's return to Sheila's case and see how a counselor might handle the disclosure process.

Counselor: "Sheila, I appreciate you keeping our appointment today. I just wanted to visit with you a few minutes about some of the difficulties you seem to be having here at school. It seems like you've been spending a lot of time with the assistant principal this semester. Can you tell me about that?

Sheila: "I don't have a problem. That stupid principal is the one with the problem. Just tell him to get off my case."

Counselor: "Sheila, I don't get involved with the discipline here at school. That's not my job. My job is to help students find ways to handle situations so they won't have to see the assistant principal. In talking to lots of different teenagers, I've found that many times when they are having problems with their grades, talking back to teachers, and fighting with other students, there is usually something going on that causes all that behavior. I'd like to know if there's anything going on that I might be able to help you with."

Sheila: "Even if there was something to talk about, you couldn't help me."

Counselor: "I don't know if I could help you or not, but I've worked with students before when they had some pretty tough problems. Why don't you give me a chance and let's see what we can work out?"

Sheila: "This is too bad for you to help with. Besides, you'd tell everybody about it."

Counselor: "It might be pretty bad, and I might have to tell someone else. Let me explain when I would have to tell someone else. If you told me that you were going to hurt yourself or somebody else, I'd have to tell someone else to keep you or the other person safe. I'd also have to tell other people if someone was physically or sexually abusing you because you might not be safe. If I did have to tell someone else, I'd tell you first that I was going to talk to someone else about what you told me, so you would always know what was going to happen."

Sheila: "I had this friend and her dad was abusing her and she told her school counselor, and he told the police and everybody else. My friend's parents got mad at her because she told and then the police took her away and put her in some home for abused kids. That counselor just created a mess for her. He didn't help her at all."

Counselor: "I can understand how that seems like a bad situation for your friend. If I had been the counselor, I would have told child protective services and the police might have gotten involved. When teenagers report to a counselor that they are being abused, the counselor must call child protective services. Usually child protective services sends out a caseworker to interview the teenager and his or her parents. Parents usually know that their teenager has reported the abuse. In some cases, the social worker may decide the child needs to leave the home at least for a while. In other cases, the social worker may decide the family needs to visit with a counselor or that the person who is hurting the teenager needs to leave the home so the teenager can stay. Even if the teenager leaves the home, he or she may go live with a relative rather than in a group home. Even though I know all that can happen, I would have reported the abuse just like the other counselor because at least your friend isn't being abused now."

This dialogue demonstrates several techniques used to explore sexual violence with a teenager. The techniques used demonstrate several steps that can be taken to encourage disclosure.

1. *Indicate an awareness of problem behaviors or physical symptoms.* The counselor introduced the idea that he or she was aware of the disciplinary problems, but was not part of the disciplinary process in the school. The counselor also used the disciplinary problems as an opportunity to explore the possibility of underlying causes. In some cases, a teacher may suspect the teenager is being abused and may refer him or her to the counselor. In this case, the counselor should just state that a teacher is concerned about the student and tell the student what behaviors or symptoms concern the teacher. However, the counselor should not indicate that the teacher suspects abuse.

2. *Use general questioning about inappropriate behaviors or physical symptoms.* Counselors should not tell the student that they think the student is being abused or even ask if the student has experienced sexual abuse, incest, or rape. Direct questioning about sexual

abuse or rape is considered to be leading the client to make allegations. Instead, the counselor should give the student the chance
to indicate that he or she is experiencing or has experienced sexual
abuse by asking general questions like the following:

> "You seem to be very angry. Can you explain to me why you are
> so angry?"
>
> "Your teacher is concerned about these behaviors. Can you tell me
> why you are acting this way?"
>
> "Sometimes behaviors (or physical symptoms) like this are related
> to situations outside the classroom. Is anything happening
> in your life that would explain these behaviors (or physical
> symptoms)?"

3. *Beware of statements that may allude to sexual abuse or violence.*
Rather than directly revealing information about sexual abuse,
incest, or rape, teenagers frequently will make indirect references
to the problem and wait to see if the counselor picks up on the
hints. Teenagers may also make references about a "friend" who
has experienced sexual violence, rather than directly discuss their
own experiences. In addition, students may make references like
the following:

> "If I told you what was happening, you wouldn't believe me."
>
> "I'm not going to talk to you or anybody else because nobody
> really knows what's going on."

4. *Be honest about the limitations of confidentiality.* Teenagers will
test you to determine if you are trustworthy. Trustworthiness
evolves from being honest with teenagers even when they don't
want to hear what you have to say and by keeping your promises
to them. Teenagers may say to you, "If I tell you this, you have to
promise me that you won't tell anyone else." Don't promise a
teenager that you will keep information confidential before you
know what they are going to tell you. You need to respond with a
statement such as, "I can't promise you that I won't tell anyone

because I don't know what you are going to tell me. I can promise you that I will try to help you deal with whatever is happening and then I'll tell you if I'm going to tell someone. If you tell me that you are being abused in some way or are going to hurt yourself or someone else, then I may have to tell someone else."

5. *Allow teenagers to disclose at their own pace.* In all likelihood, Sheila will not disclose abuse the first time she visits with a counselor. In fact, she may visit with the counselor several times and want to talk about a "friend's" situation rather than her own situation. If she decides to trust the counselor, she will disclose when she thinks she has enough information about the conse quences of the disclosure. During the process, counselors may decide to notify social services prior to the disclosure if they suspect the teenager is being abused. A word of caution here. The teenager may actually be talking about a friend and trying to persuade his or her friend to come talk with the counselor, so do not make any hasty assumptions. Before making a referral to a social service agency or the police, tell the student what action you are taking and why you are taking that action.

6. *Make a commitment to the student.* Decide you are willing to meet with the student several times and expend effort establishing a relationship. The student may need to talk with you over a period of time before he or she feels comfortable enough to disclose. Recognize that if the student has experienced sexual abuse or rape, the sexual offender may have threatened the student with state- ments like "If you tell, I'll tell everyone that you were the one who started it," "I love you, so I'm not going to tell what you have done," "Who would take your word over mine? They'll call you a liar," or "If you tell, we'll both go to jail." Although teenagers may want out of the abusive situation, they may not feel that others will see them as victims. As a result, the student may feel guilty or may feel like a partner in the sexual activity. You have to be willing to make a commitment to do whatever you can to explore what is troubling the student. At times it may be tempting to ignore the indications you see that suggest sexual violence. However, students

exhibiting symptoms of sexual abuse need a trustworthy adult to assist them in disclosing the abuse.

Dealing With Disclosure

Disclosing abuse is a difficult process for any individual who has experienced it. Teens who have experienced sexual abuse may fear that adults will not believe them or that they will be viewed as sexually promiscuous. If the abuser is an individual of the same sex, teens could fear that others will think they are gay or lesbian. Perhaps the overriding issue for teens in disclosing abuse is whether they will be accepted by others. Because of this concern about acceptance, teens may initially disclose partial information about sexual abuse to determine if the counselor is responsive. If teens feel safe disclosing to the counselor, then over a period of several sessions they will gradually disclose the full extent of the abuse. For example, teens might initially reveal that an adult has kissed them or fondled them to determine how the counselor will respond to this information. If teens perceive they are believed and accepted, then they may reveal additional information in subsequent sessions. However, counselors cannot assume a client is not revealing everything they have experienced during the initial disclosure.

Counselors have a formidable task in dealing with disclosure of sexual violence. The counselor has the dual tasks of immediately responding to the client's concerns, while at the same time maintaining accurate documentation of the client's disclosure. Returning to the counselor's interactions with Sheila will provide an example of how a counselor can be accepting of the client while making the client aware of the limits of confidentiality and of how the information will be documented.

Sheila stops by the counselor's office two or three times with questions about her "friend." Each time, the counselor gives her as much information as she can and continues to allow Sheila to make contact on her own initiative. Then one afternoon Sheila drops by the counselor's office again.

Sheila:	"Do you have time to talk to me for a few minutes?"
Counselor:	"I'll make time to talk with you. Come on in and close the door."
Sheila:	"You know my friend I've been talking about? Well, all those questions haven't been about my friend."
Counselor:	"Well, if those questions haven't been about your friend, I would guess you've needed that information yourself."
Sheila:	"Yeah, sort of."
Counselor:	"I know we have talked about this several times before, but I want to be sure that you understand that if you are being abused or hurt in any way, I will tell other people in order to keep you safe."
Sheila:	"I know."
Counselor:	"Well, since you understand I may have to tell someone, I'm going to take notes about what you say and then read back what I've written, so I make sure I understand what has been happening. Why don't you tell me what's been going on?"

Once Sheila has indicated that she might disclose sexual abuse, the counselor needs to be aware of how to document the allegations. The following guidelines are provided to help you be prepared to document allegations of sexual abuse.

1. *Document allegations carefully.* Counselors need to have careful documentation about allegations. Writing down information in front of the student allows the counselor to verify the information by checking back with the student. In addition, documenting the information at the time of disclosure helps eliminate the possibility that the counselor will not be able to accurately recall details. Counselors should keep in mind that the information regarding the initial disclosure could be used in a civil or criminal court case. Often court cases may begin months or even years after the initial disclosures. By that time, a counselor needs detailed notes to recall accurately what the client reported. Written documentation should

reflect the exact statements of the client and also note that these are allegations, not statements of fact. Documenting information in front of the student also alerts the student to the seriousness of the allegations. Occasionally, students do make false allegations, and documenting the information in front of them should help deter false allegations.

2. *Get details about who, what, when, where, and how.* The counselor needs to ask the student for specific details about where the abuse occurred and when it occurred. Pinpoint as many details as possible. However, the counselor needs to be very careful not to lead the student by suggesting who might be the perpetrator. Questions should help the student remember details in regard to what has happened to them. Questions beginning with who, what, when, where, and how allow students to explain what has happened to them without leading them. You should avoid questions that begin with did, could, and do because they lead the student's responses. Students may initially disclose only a part of the abuse, so counselors should follow up with questions like "What else has happened?" and "Has anyone else been involved?"

3. *Document how the student reacted during disclosure.* Details about the student's reactions while disclosing often provide information that will help affirm allegations. Information about the student's emotional responses and the language the student uses to describe incidents of sexual abuse will help substantiate allegations. In addition, the types of details the teen remembers and how specifically they describe the incident can be crucial in determining whether the allegations will be believed by law enforcement agencies. More information about how to determine if allegations are true or false is provided later in this chapter.

4. *Understand how police and/or social service agencies deal with allegations of sexual violence.* You need to know what steps to take if a teenager reports sexual violence. If you are not familiar with how abuse or rape allegations are investigated in your state or area, contact the local police department or child protective services

and interview knowledgeable individuals concerning the process. Teenagers who have experienced sexual violence will expect you to be able to tell them what is about to happen to them. Be honest with students concerning what might happen to them, rather than minimizing the possible outcomes.

5. *Be aware of your own response to the disclosure.* Listening to students describe sexual abuse, incest, or rape is difficult. Yet it is important that you be willing to walk back through the incident with clients as they describe it. Imagine what a teenager will think if your response indicates that the incident is too horrible for you to consider. Teenagers may decide that their experiences should not be revealed at all. When a teenager does reveal memories of sexual abuse or violence to you, you need to be compassionate during their recollections and assure them that other adolescents have experienced similar types of abuse and survived.

True or False?

As a school counselor you should not take on the task of determining whether allegations of sexual abuse or violence are true. When allegations are made, you need to assume the allegations could be true and notify child protective services and/or law enforcement agencies. School counselors must allow individuals trained to assess sexual abuse survivors to determine the believability of the allegations.

However, in dealing with initial disclosures, it would be helpful for you to have a general understanding of the characteristics used to determine if allegations are true, so you can document this type of information. Remember that these are generalizations of the characteristics of how to determine if allegations are true. If you suspect a student is making false allegations, you should not take on the role of an investigator. You do not have the training to conduct an investigation, and it is not your role as a school counselor to be Columbo. Even if you suspect the allegations are false, you need to document the allegations and make a referral to child protective services and/or the police.

Typically the following characteristics are considered when determining if allegations are true or false.

1. *Memory.* Individuals who have experienced sexual abuse usually have good recall of details. They can describe what the perpetrator was wearing and where the assault took place. Even if the individual disassociates during part of the trauma, they usually have good recall of details up to a point in the assault and then may describe a period of time when they feel like they were watching themselves. In addition, individuals who have experienced sexual trauma will describe the incident from a victim's standpoint. The words the teen uses to describe the incident may change, but the facts do not change. If students have vague recall of details or change details substantially in disclosure, they may be falsely accusing someone.

2. *Language.* Students who have been sexually assaulted will typically use language appropriate for talking with their peers. They will describe a man's penis as a "cock" or "dick" rather than using the term *penis.* They may describe vaginal penetration as "he put his thing inside me." When students are disclosing abuse, you need to be careful that you do not change the language they use to describe the trauma. Use the language the client uses. Students may use language from movies or pornographic literature to make false allegations. In which case, they may be able to describe sexual activities in great detail, but they will not use an age-appropriate vocabulary. Occasionally adults may coach teens to make allegations. If students use adult language or repetitive phrasing, the allegations may be false.

3. *Reactions to disclosure.* Teens who have experienced sexual trauma are usually hesitant to describe what they have experienced. When they do describe the trauma, their emotional responses are generally intense and congruent with allegations. They will seem fearful of the abuser and ashamed of the sexual

abuse. Often, even after clients have disclosed abuse to the counselor, they can be quite resistant to telling their parents or the police. After experiencing sexual trauma, teens will typically avoid the abuser. In contrast, when teens make false allegations, they may be angry with the abuser but seem comfortable interacting with the abuser. In fact, they may even confront the abuser as a means to gain approval from others. If the allegations are false, teens will generally be willing to talk with their parents and/or the police if a counselor encourages them to disclose the allegations. Finally, if the allegations are false, the student's emotional responses will seem incongruent with the allegations. For example, the client may seem detached or unemotional.

4. *Behavior.* If teens have experienced sexual trauma, their behavior generally changes. Their behavior can become seductive and precocious, or it may become regressed and guarded, but the behavior will change. If a teen does not exhibit behavioral changes, the allegations may be false. In addition, teens who experienced sexual trauma frequently have physical complaints such as stomachaches or headaches.

5. *Motives.* Any time a student could benefit from making the allegations in some way, the allegations should be closely scrutinized. Generally, when teens disclose sexual abuse, they perceive they have a lot to lose in terms of reputation and privacy. In contrast, most students who make false allegations experience some type of benefit in making the allegations. For example, a student can make allegations as a way to get a teacher or coach fired because the student is not successful in a class or an activity.

Developing a Plan

When students disclose sexual abuse or rape, the counselor must develop an immediate plan to respond to the situation. The counselor has to determine who might be aware of the sexual abuse or rape and what steps have been taken to insure the safety of the student. In addition, the counselor needs to assess if other children or adolescents are immediately at risk and decide who should be notified to ensure the safety of both the client and other current or potential victims. In the midst of making all of these decisions about who else needs to know, the counselor needs to be attuned to the needs of the client. Sounds a bit overwhelming? Actually, by taking things one step at a time, a counselor can provide effective support for the client, develop a safety plan, and notify individuals and agencies that need to know about the situation. The following case studies will demonstrate how the following six-step model can help the counselor develop a plan of action.

1. Decide immediately what the student needs.
2. Develop a safety plan.
3. Decide whom to notify.
4. Discuss the plan with the student.
5. Allow the student to make decisions whenever possible
6. Follow up with the student and others.

Dealing With Sexual Abuse

Daquitha played basketball with her older brothers her entire life and dreamed of playing college basketball one day. When she made the varsity team as a sophomore, she was excited and eager to make a good impression on the coach. The coach invited her to his office after practice during the second week of the preseason. The coach told Daquitha that she was making excellent progress in workouts and gave her a few tips on how to improve her game and then sent her to the locker room. The after-workout chats with the coach became a regular occurrence. By the fourth week of practice, the other coaches and players didn't think it was unusual for Daquitha to stay late and shower after the other players left the locker room. The coach began to give Daquitha a ride home after workouts.

During that fourth week of practice, Daquitha was toweling off after her shower when her coach walked into the locker room. Rather than leaving immediately, the coach looked at Daquitha and made a comment about what a great body she had. The next night he entered the locker room again before Daquitha had dressed and grabbed her from behind and forced her up against the wall. The coach fondled Daquitha and told her, "Don't you tell anybody about this. If you do, no one will believe you because everyone likes me and thinks I'm a good coach. If you say anything, everyone will think you are a slut."

As the season progressed, Daquitha's after-practice "chats" with the coach continued and the coach eventually began having intercourse with Daquitha on a regular basis. Daquitha was doing well in basketball and was a starter by the end of the season.

During the spring semester, the school counselor was startled when she was helping Daquitha fill out her schedule and noticed that she did not want to participate in basketball the next school year. The counselor questioned Daquitha concerning why she did not want to participate in basketball. Daquitha initially offered several superficial excuses for not playing basketball, then began to cry suddenly and stormed out of the office.

The following week, the counselor took Daquitha out of one of her classes to discuss the schedule again. She believed something had happened that Daquitha was hesitant to share. She decided to empathetically inquire about what had changed about basketball to make her decide she that did not want to play. Daquitha began to sob and then told her about how the coach was sexually abusing her.

Counselor's Plan of Action

1. *Decide what the student needs immediately.* Counselors should ask themselves, "What does this student need from me right now?" The student may need you to validate that you believe him or her. Your acceptance of the student may help the student accept what has happened and begin to deal with his or her feelings of anger or guilt. In addition, you may need to clarify for the student who is responsible for the abuse—the perpetrator. Daquitha was frightened of how her parents would respond. She thought they might be angry with her and blame her for the sexual abuse. A counselor would need to assure Daquitha she was not "bad" and that teenagers do not make adults engage in sexual activities with them. Daquitha was also concerned that if other people found out about the allegations, they would think she was promiscuous. Daquitha

may also need to be assured that the counselor will be able to help her find a way to end the sexual abuse.

2. *Develop a safety plan.* The counselor needs to assess whether the student or other students are currently being sexually abused. Daquitha was still involved in off-season training for basketball, and the coach still found opportunities to sexually abuse her. However, there was no indication that the coach was sexually abusing any other students. The counselor would need to ensure that Daquitha would not have contact with the coach until the allegations were investigated.

3. *Decide whom to notify.* A counselor needs to be aware of state regulations and school district policies as well as ethical guidelines concerning who must be notified about acts of sexual violence. Because Daquitha's parents are not involved in the sexual abuse and are unaware it is occurring, they need to be notified. In addition, the school principal will need to be notified, particularly because the allegations involve a school employee. In most states, the counselor will be required to report the abuse to child protective services and/or the police.

4. *Discuss the plan with the student.* The counselor can alleviate some of the student's anxiety by explaining who will be notified and how that might impact the student immediately. Daquitha had specific questions about what would happen now that she had revealed she had been sexually abused. She asked how the investigation would be conducted, how or if her coach would be punished, if she would have to confront the coach about the sexual abuse, if she would have to talk to the police, and what her coach would do when he found out that Daquitha had talked. The counselor would need to tell Daquitha that her parents, the principal, and the police must be notified.

5. *Allow the student to make decisions whenever possible.* Teenagers who have experienced sexual abuse or rape often feel a loss of control about future actions. To help empower these students,

counselors should allow them to make as many decisions as possible concerning how their parents, the school administration, the police and/or social services will be notified. A counselor could give Daquitha the option of telling her parents by herself or having the counselor present when she tells them. The counselor should prepare Daquitha for how her parents might respond to allegations of sexual abuse. Occasionally, parents may deny the situation and refuse to address the sexual abuse. If the parents do believe the allegations, they may feel guilt for failing to protect their child and/or anger at the perpetrator for hurting their child. The child may interpret these parental responses as anger toward the child or disappointment with the child. Similarly, the counselor should allow Daquitha to decide if she wants to talk with the school principal and the police herself or if she wants the counselor to make the initial report. The counselor needs to discuss with Daquitha the probability that even if the school counselor makes the initial report, there likely will be an investigation of the allegations, and she will probably have to talk with investigators at a later time.

6. *Follow up with the student and others.* The counselor will need to follow up with the student to make sure that the student is safe and is receiving adequate support from family members and professionals. The counselor may need to refer the student to a local social service agency or a counselor in private practice, to give the student an opportunity to address issues in depth that are related to sexual abuse and/or rape. Additionally, the counselor may have to provide information and/or testimony for social service agencies and the police. In Daquitha's case, her parents arranged for her to meet with a local therapist in private practice. The coach was placed on administrative leave during the investigation and eventually faced criminal charges for his actions.

Dealing With Incest

For as long as José could remember, he lived with terror. He dreaded his stepfather's order to go back to his bedroom. After José entered the bedroom, his stepfather locked the door and anally penetrated José. As José grew older, his stepfather invited his friends to engage in sexual activities with José. José's stepfather also forced José to sexually molest his younger sisters.

If José refused to engage in sexual interactions with his stepfather, his stepfather would hit him until he complied. José began to believe that he would grow up to be just like his stepfather and that he, too, would molest his children. José also wondered if he was gay because he had engaged in sexual activities with other males.

As a result of José's history of sexual abuse, he was angry and violent in his interactions with his peers and teachers. The principal referred him to the school counselor for an assessment to determine if he should be placed in a special program for emotionally disturbed adolescents. When José initially started working with the counselor, the two developed a behavior management plan for school. The counselor met with José five times before he gradually began to tell the counselor more about his home life. Over a period of several weeks, José revealed more details about his family, until he finally revealed how his stepfather physically and sexually assaulted him.

Counselor's Plan of Action

1. *Decide what the client needs immediately.* José initially was frightened about how his stepfather would respond to his allegations. He feared that his stepfather might kill him. The counselor assured José that a plan would be developed to protect him. In addition, the counselor assured José that he was not to blame for the abuse and that it was his parents' responsibility to keep him safe. The counselor told José that he would do everything possible to stop the abuse. Notice that the counselor did not promise the abuse would stop—the promise was that he would do everything he could to stop the abuse. Trustworthiness is significantly damaged when a promise is broken.

2. *Develop a safety plan.* In this case, the counselor considered José's safety and the safety of any other children living in the household. The counselor developed an immediate safety plan for José and his siblings. In most states, a counselor is required to notify child

protective services, and that agency would decide whether to immediately remove José and his siblings from the home. If José was not removed from the home, the counselor needed to help José make arrangements to spend the night at a friend's house.

3. *Decide whom to notify.* In José's situation, child protective services would need to be notified and possibly the police, depending on the state's requirements. The counselor should not notify a noncustodial parent of the allegations. The counselor should allow child protective services or the judicial system to notify the non-custodial parent. In addition, the counselor needs to be aware of school policies about notifying school administrators. In some school districts, counselors are required to tell administrators when they are reporting suspected abuse or neglect. Notification of school administration does not obviate the counselor's responsibility to notify child protective services. In most states, the counselor will be held responsible for notifying child protective services, even if the school administrator indicates he or she will notify child protective services. If the school administrator is required by school policy to be the individual who notifies child protective services, then the counselor should be present when the administrator notifies child protective services.

4. *Discuss the plan with the student.* The counselor should let José know that child protective services will be notified concerning the allegations and explain how the allegations will be investigated. Realistically, José may be removed from his home because his stepfather lives in the home. If José is removed from the home, he may feel that he is being punished while his stepfather is totally evading punishment. The counselor should also let José know if the police or a school administrator will be notified.

5. *Allow the student to make decisions whenever possible.* In José's case, there are few decisions that he can make. The counselor might give him the option to call child protective services if school policies permit this. If José indicates that he wants to contact child protective services, then the counselor needs to be present when

he notifies child protective services. Similarly, the counselor might allow José to choose where he wants to wait for the police or social workers from child protective services.

6. *Follow up with the student and others.* If José was removed from his home, the counselor might contact child protective services and/or the police to verify that interventions had been taken to ensure José's safety. If José was left in his home, the counselor could meet with him to see that support and assistance were being provided. In addition, if José remains in the home, the counselor might need to contact his mother to help make arrangements for José to receive long-term counseling services from a local social service agency or a private practitioner who understands the issues of incest survivors. Child protective services can assist in arranging for counseling services because they have knowledge and frequent contact with counselors who work with incest survivors.

Dealing With Date Rape

Kendra, a sophomore, had not dated much, so she was excited when William began to spend time with her. After attending three school activities together, William asked Kendra to come watch a movie at Chad's house. William assured Kendra that it would be fun and that Chad and his girlfriend, Anna, would be there. William also told Kendra that Chad's parents would be at home as well.

When Kendra and William went to Chad's house, the two couples went to the basement to watch the movie while Chad's parents remained upstairs. Not long after the movie started, Chad and Anna started "making out." Kendra felt awkward, but kept watching the movie while trying to ignore Chad and Anna. A little bit later, Chad and Anna got up and went into one of the bedrooms in the basement.

Kendra and William continued to watch the movie without comment. William put his arm around Kendra and began kissing her. Kendra initially was excited, but as William's actions became more intimate, Kendra told him to stop several times. William put his hand over Kendra's mouth and said, "Don't you tell me to stop. You've wanted me to do this all evening."

Kendra struggled to get away from William, but he used his body to pin her to the couch. When Kendra started to scream, William told her, "Shut up, or I will really hurt you."

After William raped Kendra, he straightened his clothes and began watching the movie as though nothing had happened. Kendra numbly pulled her clothes back on and sat watching the movie again.

When Kendra got home that night, she wondered if she had not made it clear enough to William that she did not want to have sex with him. She berated herself for agreeing to go to Chad's house because she thought she should have realized that William wanted her to have sex with him. Kendra thought back on several inter-actions she had with William and began to think she should have recognized what was going to happen before it happened.

Kendra saw William several times at school the next day, and he continued to act as though nothing had happened the previous night. As Kendra sat in class that day, she worried about whether she could be pregnant. By the last class period of the day, she decided to talk to the school counselor to find out if she might be pregnant. In discuss-ing the situation with the school counselor, Kendra stated that she had repeatedly asked William to stop, but he refused to stop.

Counselor's Plan of Action

1. *Decide what the student needs immediately.* Kendra is anxious and concerned that she might be pregnant. In addition, she feels guilty about placing herself in a situation where she could be raped. She is blaming herself rather than William and assuming that she "asked for it." The counselor should help Kendra clarify her role in the situation by using questions like "When you agreed to go to Chad's house, did you think you were going there to have sex?" "Did you ask William to stop?" and "Did you want to have sex with William last night?" The counselor should help Kendra rec-ognize that when she said "No" and William continued, she did not consent to sexual activity. The counselor may also need to address Kendra's concerns about pregnancy.

2. *Develop a safety plan.* Kendra should recognize that she need not date William and that he might attempt to rape her again if she

continues to do so. Kendra may need to elicit her parents' support in helping her set boundaries.

3. *Decide whom to notify.* The counselor may be required by school policy to notify a school administrator and may be required by state law to notify Kendra's parents and/or the police. In addition, the counselor may want to contact the local rape crisis agency and make arrangements for Kendra to meet with a counselor.

4. *Discuss the plan with the student.* The counselor should explain applicable school policies and state laws to Kendra. The option of contacting the rape crisis center should also be presented to Kendra

5. *Allow the student to make decisions when possible.* It is possible that the counselor is not required by school policy or state law to contact anyone about date rape. If this is the case, Kendra should decide who she would want to know about the rape. Kendra may be anxious about telling her parents and/or the police. The counselor should explore with Kendra the possible positive and negative consequences of telling her parents and/or the police. If the counselor is required by school policy or state law to report the rape, then the student should be given the option of being present during those disclosures if possible.

6. *Follow up with the student and others.* The counselor should meet with Kendra again to see if she is getting the support and intervention services she needs. If the counselor contacted the rape crisis center, he or she may need to make a follow-up contact to see that the student is receiving services.

Dealing With Stranger Rape

Sherri arrived at school half an hour late and was crying when she came to the office to get a tardy pass for class. When the attendance clerk asked why Sherri was late to class, Sherri began crying even harder. The attendance clerk was concerned, so she called the school counselor. The school counselor took Sherri into her office.

Once Sherri calmed down, she was able to tell the counselor why she was crying. Sherri told the counselor that she had been walking to school like she did every morning. As Sherri started to cross the street, a car pulled around the corner and blocked her way across the street. A man jumped from the car and pulled Sherri into the car. After the driver of the car pulled into the alley, both men in the car raped Sherri and then shoved her out of the car. The men drove down the alley and Sherri numbly returned to her routine and walked to school.

After recounting the incident, Sherri assured the counselor that she would feel much better if she could just take a shower and put on some different clothes.

Counselor's Plan of Action

1. *Decide what the student needs immediately.* Sherri is still in shock from the trauma of being raped and needs to be assured that she is safe. However, she should not be allowed to take a shower and change clothes because that will destroy crucial evidence of the crime. The counselor should help Sherri feel comfortable in her office and encourage her to stay in the office until one of her parents can be contacted.

2. *Develop a safety plan.* Sherri is in no immediate danger.

3. *Decide whom to notify.* The rape crisis center, the police, and Sherri's parents all have to be notified immediately. School policy may also require that the counselor notify a school administrator.

4. *Discuss the plan with the student.* The counselor should let Sherri know who is being contacted and why they are being contacted. The counselor should let Sherri know that typically a rape exam is done at the hospital to ensure her health and to help gather evidence. The information should be presented in a calm, matter-of-fact way so that it does not create more anxiety for Sherri.

5. *Allow the student to make decisions whenever possible.* If Sherri is calm enough, she should be given the option of calling her parents, the police, and the rape crisis center. However, she should be assured that the counselor will handle these tasks if asked.

6. *Follow up with the student and others.* After the initial crisis intervention, the counselor should contact the student to help her make the transition to returning to school. Sherri's parents may also need a referral for counseling at the rape crisis center or with a counselor in private practice. The counselor should follow up by contacting the rape crisis center and the police.

What About the Counselor?

There are three primary issues for the counselor in dealing with sexual violence. The first issue is to determine areas of skill and competency. Generally, school counselors do not have the training, skills, or time available that is necessary to deal with long-term individual counseling for victims of sexual abuse. Instead, school counselors may provide the immediate response and crisis intervention needed to help students. Then the counselor's role is to help the student gain access to available support services in local social service agencies or through private practitioners. If school counselors find themselves dealing with issues beyond their competency and skills, they need to make a referral or find someone with the needed expertise to provide consultation or supervision.

The second issue for counselors who deal with sexual violence is the personal effect of listening to accounts of sexual trauma. Recognize that hearing students tell of their experiences with sexual violence may be emotionally draining and leave counselors numb for a period of time. Counselors may reexperience traumatic incidents or even have nightmares about the trauma. Counselors cannot avoid being affected by hearing the pain and fear that a student has experienced while being sexually traumatized. Counselors may even find that they question the fairness and predictability of their own world.

Counselors must find ways to deal with how disclosures of trauma affect them. Counselors may need to process their responses with another counselor or keep a journal about their reactions. Perhaps listening to quiet music or taking a walk through a park will be a soothing experience to help counselors process what has happened to them. Regardless of what counselors do to deal with their reactions to hearing about sexual violence, they need to attend to that response in some fashion.

In dealing with sexual violence, a third issue for counselors is their personal issues about sexual violence. Counselors who have experienced rape, incest, or sexual abuse need to be extremely aware of how their personal experiences with sexual violence affect the way they interact with clients who have experienced sexual violence. Counselors cannot work effectively with clients who have experienced sexual violence if they have not worked through their own issues. Counselors who have not dealt with their personal experiences with sexual violence may allow countertransference to interfere with the client's issues. If counselors have not worked through their own issues about sexual violence, ethically they must refer clients who are dealing with sexual violence to another counselor.

Summary

Recognize that if you are effective in your interventions as a school counselor, you may help end a cycle of sexual violence. When a teenager has experienced sexual violence, he or she is likely to enter into other relationships with similar characteristics unless some intervention occurs. Teenagers often may believe that the sexual violence is deserved and have a self-concept based on the premise that only "bad" people experience sexual violence. With this underlying premise, teenagers may then internalize the idea that they are "bad" and deserve to be abused or neglected. Teenagers who have experienced neglect or abuse may have feelings of foreboding concerning the future and may believe that death is inevitable before reaching adulthood.

With effective counseling and intervention, teenagers who have experienced sexual trauma will form healthy relationships with others and make sexuality decisions based on a healthy self-concept. In addition, sexually traumatized teenagers can learn that other teenagers have survived sexual trauma; and as a result, they will envision a future without sexual violence.

5

Dare to Dream

In writing this book, we hope to have challenged school counselors to be more effective in helping teens deal with sexual issues. We hope that a counselor like Lynn Adams in Chapter 1 will be willing to tackle the tough sexual issues that teens bring to them. We are convinced that at some time in counselors' careers, they decide to help teens address sexual issues, or they gradually shut themselves off from teens by ignoring or minimizing sexual concerns voiced by students. The challenge for counselors is to face their own emotional reactions to sexual issues and to learn effective ways to intervene with adolescents. Let's return to a discussion of Lynn Adams. Here is what we hope would happen after Lynn recognized the types of sexual issues teens are confronted with daily.

When Lynn clearly understood what she believed about sexuality, she began to reconceptualize her role as a school counselor. Lynn understood that teens needed more from her than just occasional advice. As a school counselor, she needed to function in a variety of roles if she was going to address the sexuality concerns of teens. Although some of these concerns would be addressed through individual counseling sessions, the most effective avenues for addressing teen sexuality would require involving students, teachers, school nurses, parents, and community agencies. Developing a comprehensive approach to addressing teen sexuality demanded that Lynn clearly understand school policies about sexuality. Lynn scheduled appointments to talk with both the school district's guidance director and her school's principal. Lynn asked questions about the school district's policy for handling sexuality issues. She obtained written guidelines for reporting sexual abuse or rape, for handling allegations of sexual harassment, and for presenting students with information about sexually transmitted diseases and birth control methods. Once Lynn was familiar with the school district's policies, she began to formulate a plan for addressing some of the sexual issues with which her students struggled. Lynn detailed the steps she would take and then met again with her principal and guidance director to confirm that her strategies complied with school policies.

Lynn's strategy for addressing sexual issues involved several steps. First, she recognized the need to educate teachers so that they would be more aware of some of the sexual concerns of adolescents. She set up a series of inservice trainings for teachers with the goal of helping teachers recognize when adolescents might need to be referred to a counselor to discuss sexual concerns. The first inservice training outlined symptoms of sexual violence and emphasized how sexual violence might be manifested in behavioral changes in the classroom or a change in academic performance. The second inservice training outlined types of behaviors and comments that constituted sexual harassment, the school's role in preventing sexual harassment of students, and specific strategies teachers could use to discourage sexual harassment. A third inservice training addressed how gay and lesbian students experience discrimination and harassment in school and ways to prevent these behaviors. A final inservice training presented information about ways to incorporate effective strategies for addressing teen pregnancy and sexually transmitted diseases across the curriculum.

In addition to providing inservice training for teachers, Lynn began to offer informational sessions for parents. Lynn scheduled sessions twice a month. She presented one session a month in the evening and one session a month on a Saturday morning. Both of these sessions covered the same material, but Lynn was able to involve more parents by having two options for attending the session. The informational sessions initially focused on helping parents develop a greater awareness of the pressures teenagers face about sexuality. Lynn used excerpts from movies and television programs to help parents understand how much sexuality affects their children's views of themselves in adolescence. After some initial sessions to emphasize the importance of developing an awareness of teen sexuality, Lynn presented more specific information about ways parents can talk with their teens and help their teens deal with sexual issues. Lynn was surprised that parents attended these sessions regularly and participated in developing parent support groups.

In addition to involving teachers and parents, Lynn involved community members and agencies. She visited local community agencies and developed a referral list that detailed the agency's address, phone number, and services available to students. She also located several community members who were willing to donate time to speak in a variety of classes, and she developed a list of these community members, ways to contact them, and topics they would address for different classes. When possible, she tried to hear these community members speak and outlined for teachers the approaches they used to address topics so that teachers could more effectively decide whether the community member would be an appropriate speaker for their courses. She distributed this list to teachers in her school and encouraged them to provide feedback on the quality of presentations the community members provided.

Lynn recognized that if students were going to approach her about discussing sexual issues, they first would have to perceive that she was willing to discuss sexuality. One of the most effective ways for Lynn to reach a large number of students was through classroom guidance activities. When Lynn had previously tried to present guidance activities to teens, she found they were often inattentive and resistant to participating. She realized that her previous guidance presentations had primarily lectured about the dangers of sexual activities. When Lynn began to emphasize participatory activities in her guidance presentations, the students were more attentive and more involved in the process. Lynn actually found that she looked forward to guidance presentations rather than dreading them.

In addition to changing her approach to guidance presentations, Lynn began to form a number of support groups in the school about sexual issues. Lynn knew three or four of her female students had experienced sexual violence, so she invited them to participate in a support group for survivors of sexual violence. Each of those students agreed to attend an initial meeting about the support group. Lynn also posted an announcement on her door about the support group. She was surprised when seven students attended the initial meeting for the support group. Gradually, she began keeping a list of names of additional students who would be interested in starting another support group. Students seemed to get information about the group primarily from other students. As the school year progressed, students expressed an interest in starting support groups for gay and lesbian students and for male survivors of sexual violence.

Involving students, teachers, parents, and community members in a variety of programs and activities helped Lynn reach out to a larger number of students than individual counseling allowed. However, Lynn was most surprised at how differently students interacted with her in individual counseling sessions. Lynn began to invite students to talk more about sexual issues, and she found that students were willing, and even eager at times, to discuss sexual issues with her once they recognized that she would be comfortable talking about them. Lynn recognized that students had not been as willing to discuss their sexual concerns with her before because of her own discomfort with talking about sexuality. She had allowed her discomfort to create a barrier between herself and the students in talking about sexual issues. After exploring her own feelings about sexuality and becoming comfortable with her own values, Lynn no longer felt uncomfortable talking about sexual issues, and students recognized that she would be comfortable talking with them.

Cautions and Dangers

Admittedly, Lynn would encounter many barriers and difficult situations in developing the skills and support systems needed to help students deal with sexual concerns. Lynn, like any counselor, could get in trouble addressing sexual issues with teenagers. Because adults often are uncomfortable with sexual issues, they may be suspicious of counselors who are at ease in talking about sexuality with teenagers. The counselor may be perceived as seductive or inappropriate if he or she discusses sexual issues with students. To help prevent or reduce allegations of seductiveness or inappropriateness, counselors should be professional in their approach to handling sexual issues and should set appropriate professional boundaries with students. Students may become infatuated with a counselor and begin to shift the boundaries of the relationship. If this occurs, the counselor should consult with another professional counselor for supervision or make a referral to another counselor.

Another difficulty counselors may encounter in addressing teen sexual issues is that administrators and/or parents may criticize or censor the counselor's activities. Parents, teachers, and administrators may believe that sexual issues should be discussed at home or by clergy rather than discussed by school counselors, particularly in conservative communities. They may actually think that discussing sexual issues causes teens to think more about sexual activities and thus encourages teens to engage in more sexual activities. Although there will always be parents and administrators who criticize any attempts to address sexual issues, counselors can address these concerns by educating parents and administrators about the types of sexual issues and problems teens struggle with today. In addition, the counselor can address criticism by providing a rationale for the programs and activities they use to discuss sexual issues in the school.

One final word of caution for counselors who are addressing sexual issues with teens. Counselors need to be aware of their own values and beliefs about sexual issues and be aware of ways to set appropriate boundaries with students. Students will be harmed rather than helped if counselors are getting their own needs met rather than focusing on the students' needs in the counseling relationship. In addition, counselors should recognize that it is not ethical for them to promote their own values rather than to accept the values of the student in a counseling relationship. Values are inherent in working with sexual issues and counselors should be respectful of their students' values. That is not to say counselors cannot help students clarify the values they are basing decisions on, but it is not the counselor's job to force students to accept the counselor's value system.

The Challenge

A recurring theme in this book is to expect the adolescent to expect more from you. The reason? Adolescents are more open with their thoughts and questions than were adolescents 25 years ago. In the past, a common response to sexual concerns and/or questions was to ignore them, act embarrassed, or say "go ask someone else." Our challenge to you, the school counselor, is to help adolescents deal with sexual concerns. Counselors who ignore the importance of sexuality in the lives of adolescents miss an opportunity to develop relationships with teens and to help them develop healthy boundaries and relationships with peers. Minimizing the impact of sexuality in the lives of teens may be more comfortable for counselors, but counselors who explore their own ideas and values about sexuality allow themselves to grow personally as well as discover more effective interventions for teens. This book is about daring to dream of a school where counselors will accept the challenges of teen sexuality and will be willing to seek out training and supervision to help develop programs that meet teens where they are. No longer can we wait for teens to come to us, we must go to where the teens are in exploring their sexuality.

The values and beliefs teens have about sexuality may not be comfortable for us at times, but if we cannot accept teens where they are, we will not have any dialogue with them about sexual issues. Adolescents want more than your brains. They want to know you care and understand. If we hope for teens to begin to make appropriate, healthy choices about sexuality, we must have an attitude of acceptance and be available for them. They must have the reassurance that we will listen to them nonjudgmentally. They will never hear our words if they do not believe we accept who they are. We might not agree with a teen trying to get pregnant by a student who has two children with two other students, but we cannot begin a conversation with this teen by condemning her values. Rather, a conversation with this student begins with us listening to who she is and why she is making this choice to try to get pregnant. When she knows we are listening and trying to understand, only then will she try to listen and understand a different perspective of the situation.

In *All About Sex: The School Counselor's Guide to Handling Tough Adolescent Problems,* we have provided you with ideas to challenge the way you view teen sexuality and suggestions to help you reconceptualize your role and strategies in addressing teen sexual issues. As Figure 5.1 illustrates, we discussed such issues as body image, dating, love and romance, intercourse and abstinence, teen pregnancy and sexually transmitted diseases, gay and lesbian issues, and the violence cycle in which we focused on sexual abuse, incest, and rape.

In this book, we have focused on the links between the counselor's tackling challenging sexual issues and enhancement of the adolescent's development. The resources listed at the end of this book provide some excellent information to help you develop additional skills for working with sexual issues. In addition, we have provided illustrations via case studies and discussed their implications. Throughout the book, we have focused on the correlation between the counselor's willingness to tackle challenging sexual issues and the adolescent's positive development.

Dealing with sexual issues is a complex, difficult process that goes far beyond helping adolescents understand anatomy and physiology, and instead delves into the very nature of sexual issues. Dealing

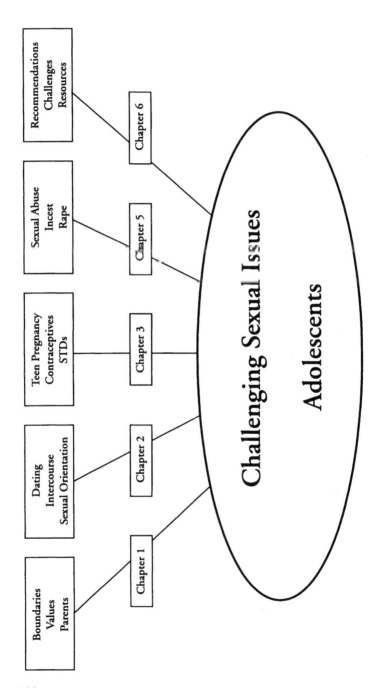

Figure 5.1 Challenging Issues

with sexual issues requires a willingness to explore how sexuality affects teens' self-concepts and their way of seeing themselves in relationships with other people. In addition, talking about sexual issues demands a willingness to consider emotional consequences of sexual activities, to discuss how decisions about sexuality affect the student's spirituality, and to consider what students' views concerning sexuality imply about their culture. What can you do to be more effective in dealing with sexual issues? As a counselor, you can

- Be an advocate for adolescents
- Care about and respond to all adolescent concerns
- Provide competent counseling to adolescents via individual and group counseling
- Educate adolescents about challenging sexual issues via classroom guidance activities
- Establish adolescent and parent support groups
- Develop a network of professional counselors for referrals as needed
- Develop a network of referral sources (e.g., agencies, health services, support services)

Although developing strategies and programs can help effectively address adolescent sexual development, do not forget the most effective tool you can provide. As a counselor you can provide the most important ingredient necessary for teens struggling to understand their developing sexuality. You can provide a relationship where it is safe to be a sexual person. If teens find a safe relationship where they can discuss their sexual concerns, they will never have to navigate their course of sexual development alone. They will have a relationship with you and your acceptance of them.

Resources

Books for Adolescents

Chapter 2

Bauer, M. D. (1995). *Am I blue? Coming out from the silence.* New York: HarperCollins Children's Books.

Bell, R. (1988). *Changing bodies, changing lives: A book for teens on sex and relationships.* New York: Vintage.

Blume, J. (1989). *Forever.* New York: Pocket Books.

Creech, S. (1997). *Absolutely normal chaos.* New York: HarperCollins Children's Books.

Crutcher, C. (1986). *Running loose.* New York: Bantam Doubleday Dell Books for Young Readers.

Crutcher, C. (1992). *Athletic shorts: Six short stories.* New York: Bantam Doubleday Dell Books for Young Readers.

Daly, M. (1985). *Seventeenth summer.* New York: Pocket Books.

Fricke, A., & Fricke, W. (1992). *Sudden strangers: The story of a gay son and his father.* New York: St. Martin's.

Garden, N. (1991). *Lark in the morning.* New York: Farrar, Straus, & Giroux.

Garden, N. (1992). *Annie on my mind.* New York: Farrar, Straus, & Giroux.

Greene, B. (1997). *The drowning of Stephan Jones.* New York: Bantam Doubleday Dell Books for Young Readers.

Guy, R. (1991). *Ruby.* New York: Dell.

Harris, R. H. (1994). *It's perfectly normal: A book about changing bodies, growing up, sex, and sexual health.* Cambridge, MA: Candlewick.

Jukes, M. (1996). *It's a girl thing: How to stay healthy, safe, and in charge.* New York: Knopf.

Kerr, M. E. (1995). *Deliver us from Evie.* New York: HarperCollins Children's Books.

Koertge, R. (1989). *The Arizona kid.* New York: Avon.

Levenkron, S. (1989). *The best little girl in the world.* New York: Warner.

Madares, L. (1988). *The what's happening to my body? Book for boys.* New York: Newmarket.

McCants, W. D. (1995). *Much ado about prom night.* San Diego: Harcourt Brace.

Newman, L. (1996). *Fat chance.* New York: Putnam.

Philbrick, R. (1995). *Freak the mighty.* New York: Scholastic.

Ripslinger, J. (1994). *Triangle.* San Diego, CA: Harcourt Brace.

Spinelli, J. (1996). *Crash.* New York: Random House of Books for Young Readers.

Stoppard, M. (1997). *Sex ed: Growing up, relationships, and sex.* New York: DK Publishing.

Thomas, R. (1996). *Rats saw God.* New York: Simon & Schuster Children's.

Woodson, J. (1997). *From the notebooks of Melanin Sun.* New York: Scholastic.

Woodson, J. (1997). *The house you pass on the way.* New York: Bantam Doubleday Dell Books for Young Readers.

Chapter 3

Christiansen, C. B. (1996). *I see the moon*. New York: Simon & Schuster Children's.

Davis, D. (1994). *My brother has AIDS*. New York: Simon & Schuster Trade.

Moore, M. (1997). *Under the mermaid angel*. New York: Bantam Doubleday Dell Books for Young Readers.

Sparks, B. (Ed.). (1994). *It happened to Nancy: A true story from the diary of a teenager*. New York: Avon.

Williams-Garcia, R. (1995). *Like sisters on the home front*. New York: Dutton Children's Books.

Wolff, Virginia E. (1995). *Make lemonade*. New York: Henry Holt.

Chapter 4

Crutcher, C. (1991). *Chinese handcuffs*. Bantam Doubleday Dell Books for Young Readers.

Hall, L. (1984). *The boy in the off-white hat*. New York: Scribners.

Hyde, M. O. (1987). *Sexual abuse: Let's talk about it*. Louisville, KY; Westminster/John Knox.

Mazer, N. F. (1994). *Out of control*. New York: Avon.

Nathanson, L. (1986). *The trouble with Wednesdays*. New York: Putman/Pacer.

Peck, R. (1977). *Are you in the house alone?* New York: Bantam Doubleday Dell Books for Young Readers.

Roberts, W. D. (1996). *Don't hurt Laurie*. Magnolia: Peter Smith.

Terkel, S. N., & Rench, J. E. (1984). *Feeling safe, feeling strong: How to avoid sexual abuse and what to do if it happens to you*. Minneapolis, MN: Lerner.

Voigt, C. (1996). *When she hollers*. New York: Scholastic.

White, R. (1994). *Weeping willow*. New York: Farrar, Straus, & Giroux.

Woodson, J. (1995). *I hadn't meant to tell you this*. New York: Bantam Doubleday Dell Books for Young Readers.

Movies/Videos for Adolescents

And the Band Played On

Angus Bethune

The Best Little Girl in the World

The Birdcage

The Breakfast Club

An Early Frost

Freak the Mighty

In and Out

In the Gloaming

The Incredibly True Story of Two Girls in Love

Perfect Body

Philadelphia

She Fought Alone

References and Suggested Readings

References

Leukefeld, C. G., & Haverkos, H. W. (1993). Sexually transmitted diseases. In T. P. Gullotta, G. R. Adams, & R. Montemayor (Eds.), *Adolescent sexuality* (pp. 161-180). Newbury Park, CA: Sage.

MacBeth, R., & Fine, N. (1995). *Playing with fire: Creative conflict resolution for young adults.* Philadelphia, PA: New Society.

Planned Parenthood. (1997). *Birth control choices for teens* [Brochure]. New York: Author.

Suggested Readings

Chapter 2

Calderone, M. S., & Ramey, J. W. (1982). *Talking with your child about sex.* New York: Ballantine.

Elkind, D. (1984). *All grown up and no place to go: Teenager in crisis.* Reading, MA: Addison-Wesley.

Heron, A. (Ed.). (1983). *One teenager in ten: Writings by gay and lesbian youth.* Boston: Alyson.

Pipher, M. (1994). *Reviving Ophelia: Saving the selves of adolescent girls.* New York: Ballantine.

Pope, K. S., Sonne, J. L., & Holroyd, J. (1993). *Sexual feelings in psychotherapy: Explorations for therapists and therapists-in-training.* Washington, DC: American Psychological Association.

Rench, J. E. (1990). *Understanding sexual identity: A book for gay and lesbian teens and their friends.* Minneapolis, MN: Lerner.

Schneider, M. (1988). *Often invisible: Counseling gay and lesbian youth.* Toronto, Canada: Central Toronto Youth Services.

Sears, J. (1991). *Growing up gay in the South: Race, gender, and journeys of the spirit.* New York: Haworth.

Woog, D. (1995). *School's out: The impact of gay and lesbian issues on America's schools.* Boston: Alyson.

Chapter 3

Gullotta, T. P., Adams, G. R., & Montemayor, R. (Eds.). (1993). *Adolescent sexuality.* Newbury Park, CA: Sage.

Jennings, C. (1988). *Understanding and preventing AIDS: A book for everyone.* Cambridge, MA: Health Alert.

Kain, C. D. (1989). *No longer immune: A counselor's guide to AIDS.* Alexandria, VA: American Association of Counseling & Development.

Simpson, C. (1996). *Coping with an unplanned pregnancy.* New York: Rosen.

Stange, J. (Ed.). (1995). *Teenagers and AIDS in America.* Commack, NY: Nova Science.

Sweets, P. W. (1995). *The art of talking with your teenager.* Holbrook, MA: Adams Media.

Chapter 4

Creighton, A., & Kivel, P. (1992). *Helping teens stop violence: A practical guide for counselors, educators, and parents.* Alameda, CA: Hunter House.

Davis, L. (1990). *The courage to heal workbook.* New York: Harper & Row.

Gil, E., & Johnson, T. C. (1993). *Sexualized children: Assessment and treament of sexualized children and children who molest.* Rockville, MD: Launch.

McBeth, F., & Fine, N. (1995). *Playing with fire: Creative conflict resolutions for young adults.* Philadelphia, PA: New Society.

Index

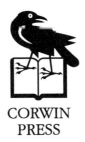

CORWIN
PRESS

The Corwin Press logo—a raven striding across an open book—represents the happy union of courage and learning. We are a professional-level publisher of books and journals for K–12 educators, and we are committed to creating and providing resources that embody these qualities. Corwin's motto is "Success for All Learners."

R